BEACH DOGS

A No Text Picture Book

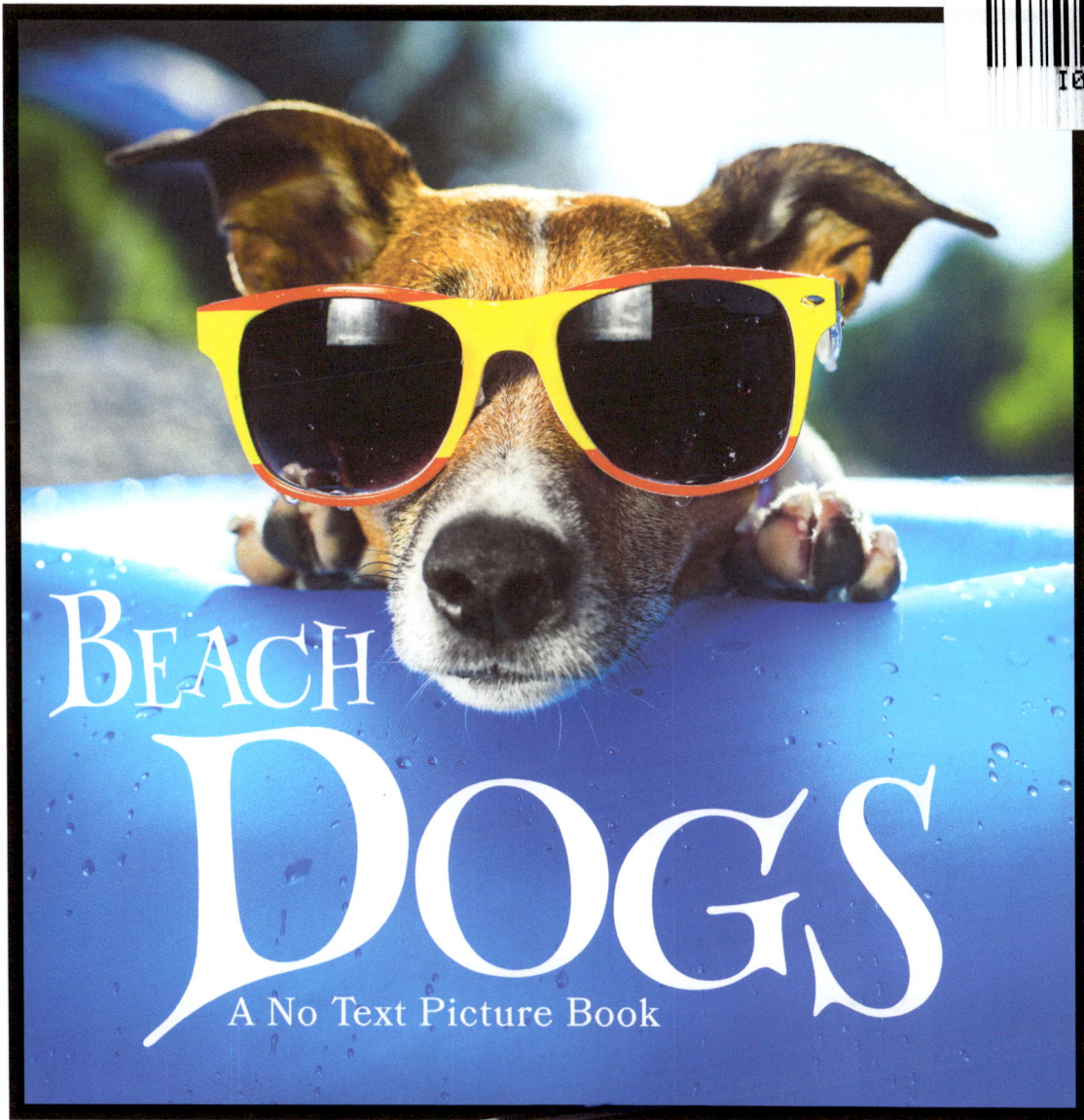

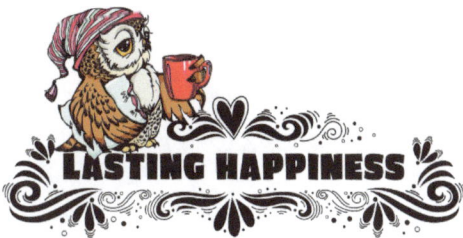

© 2020 Lasting Happiness | All rights reserved.
No part of this book may be reproduced or copied in any manner without prior written permission from the publisher.

ISBN: 978-1-990181-21-4

LASTING HAPPINESS

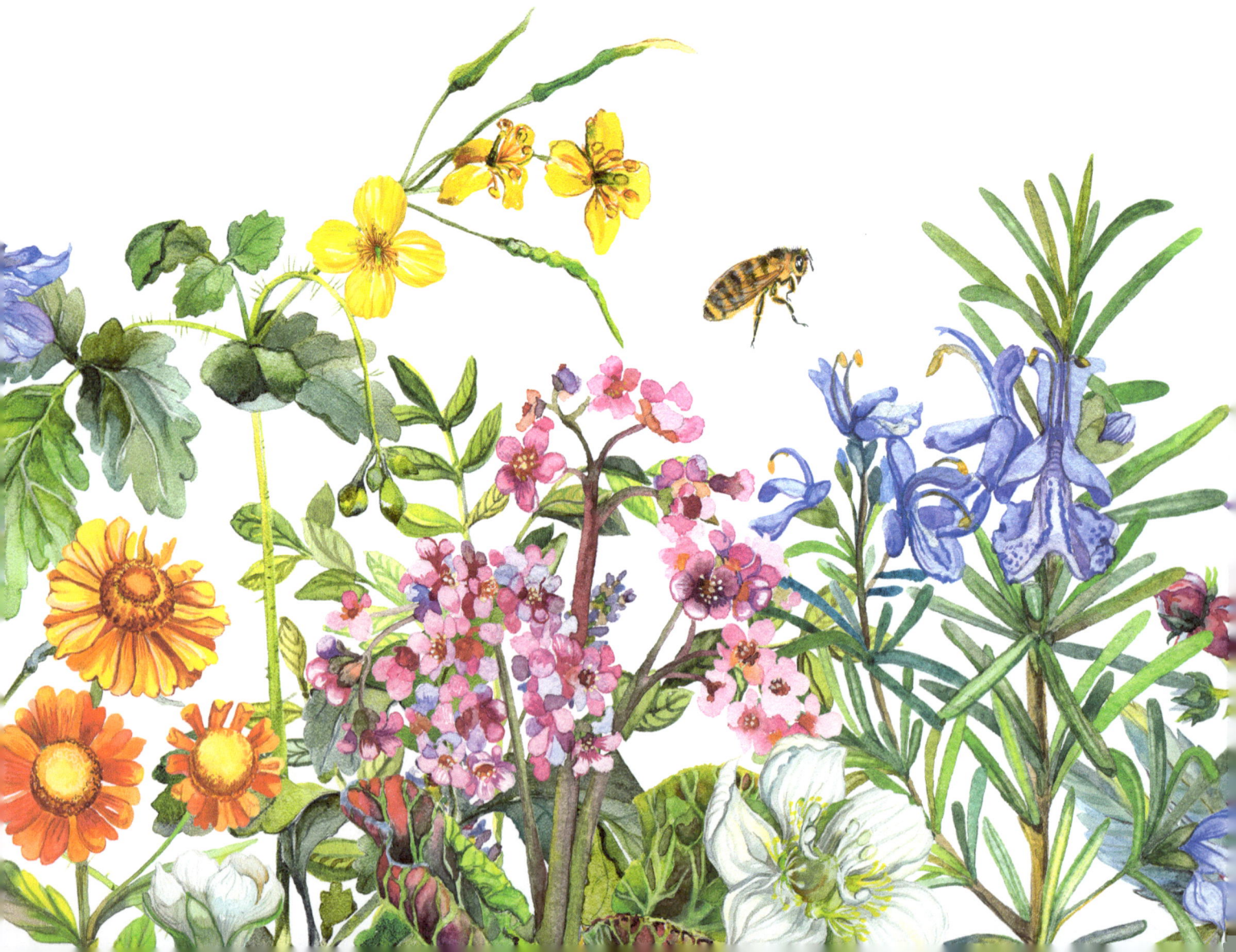

To:

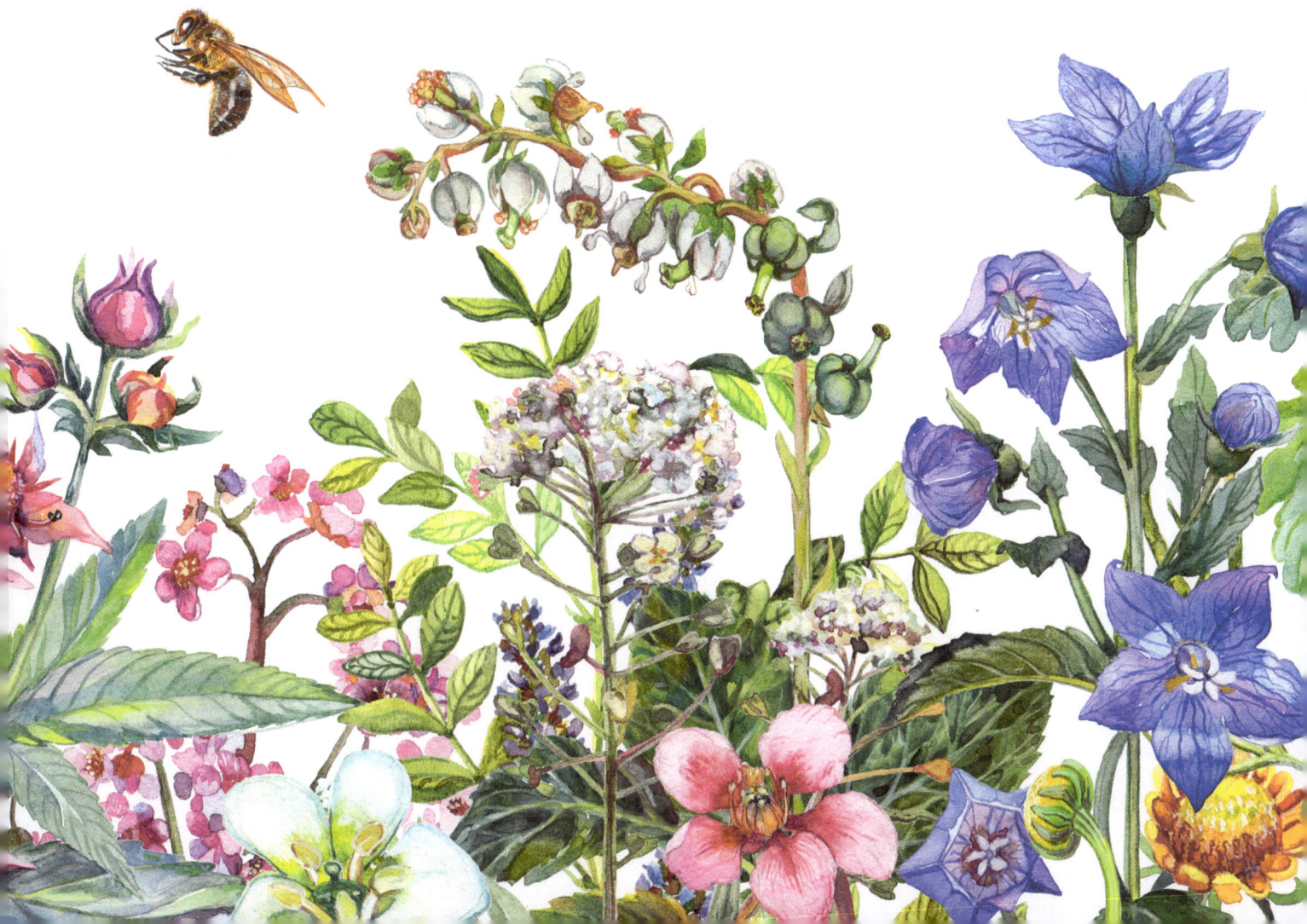

FROM:

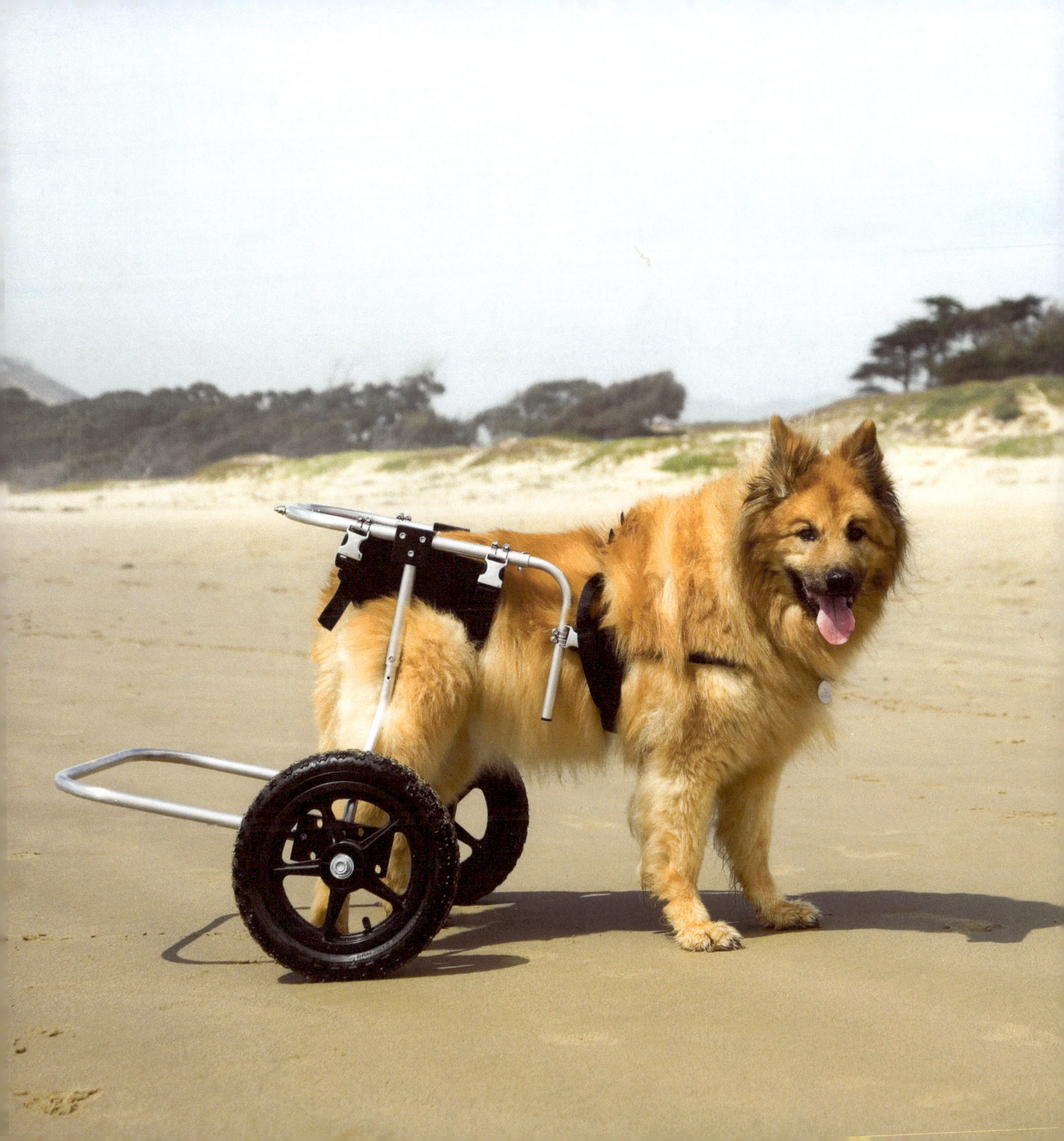

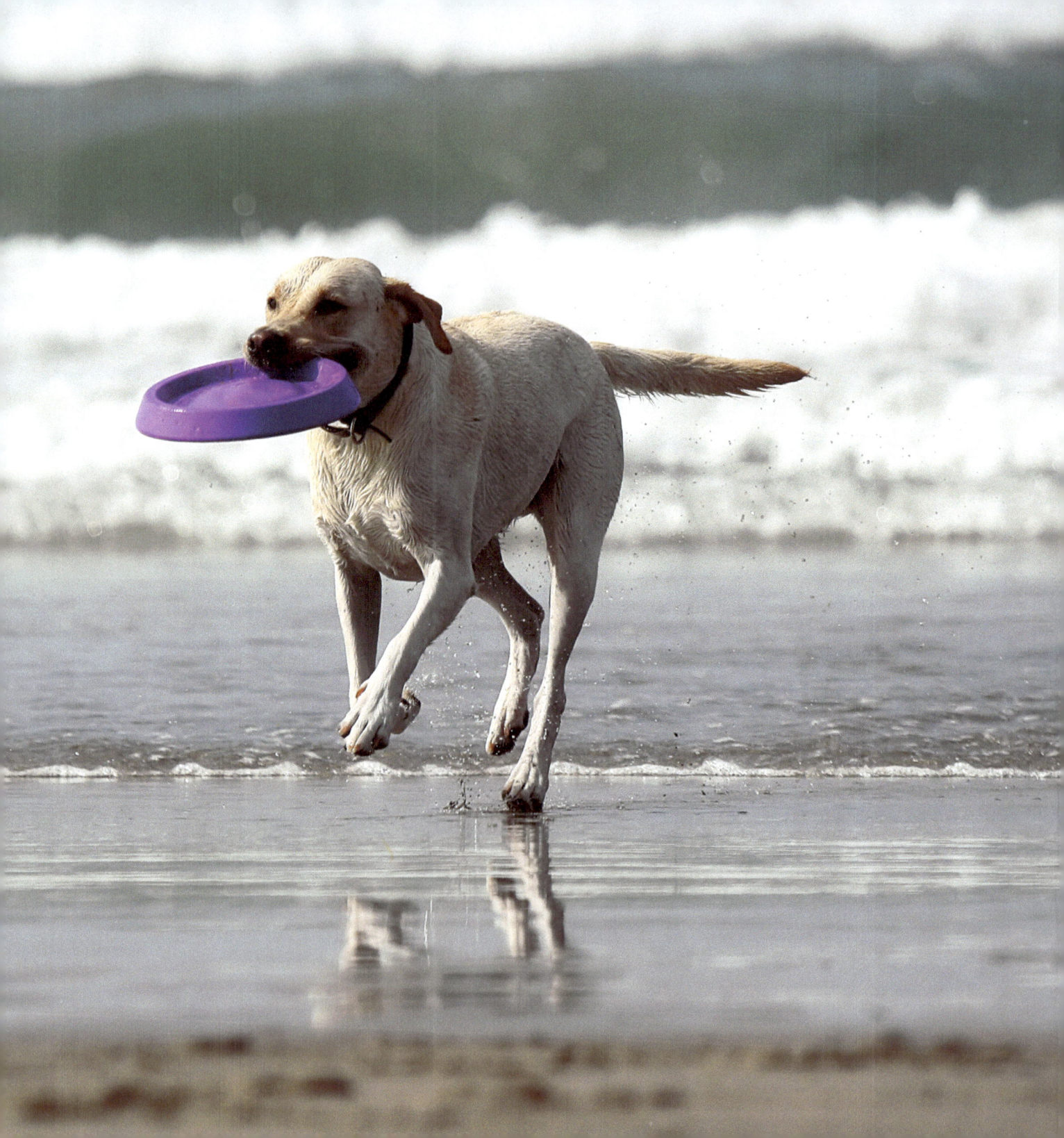

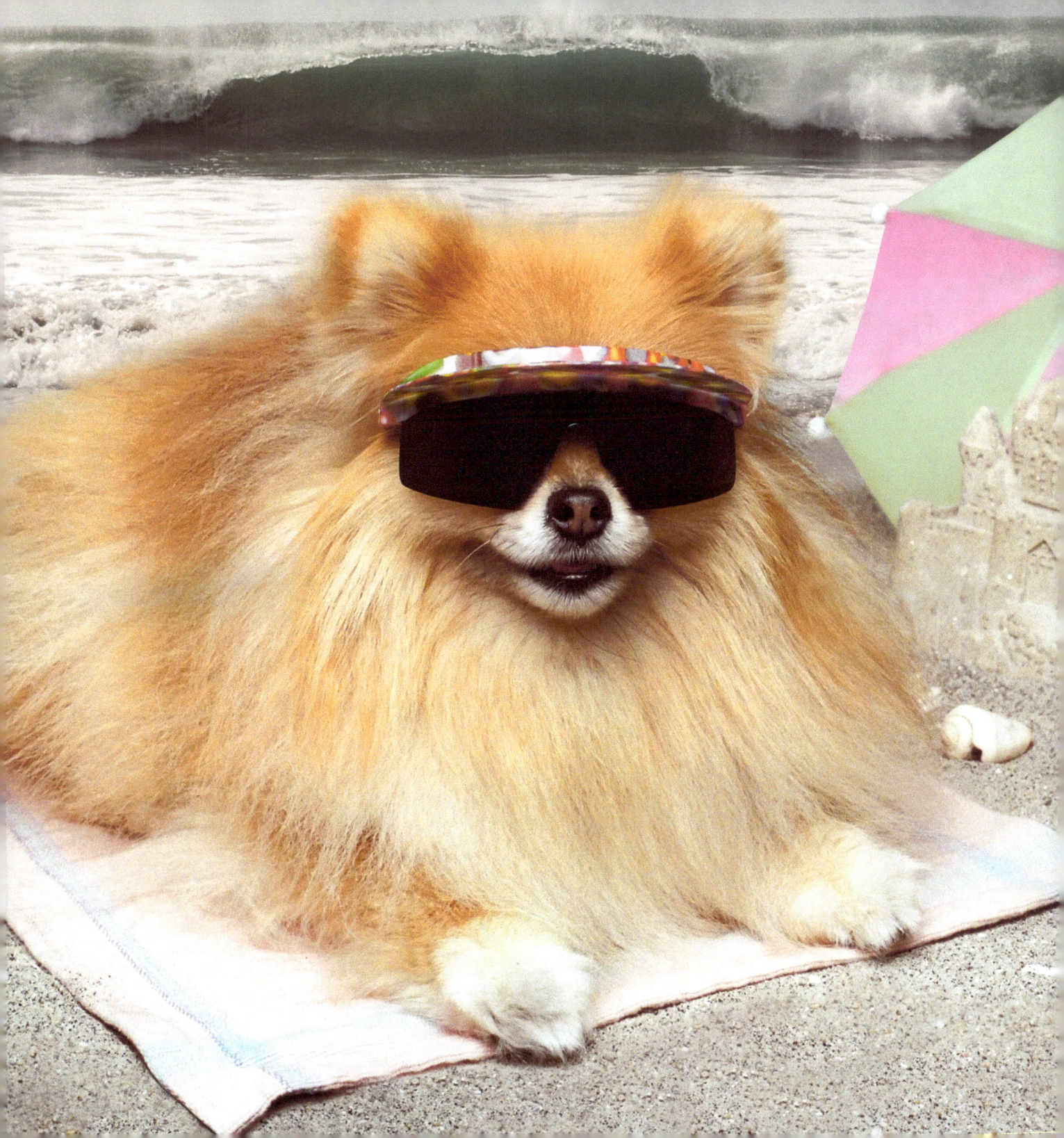

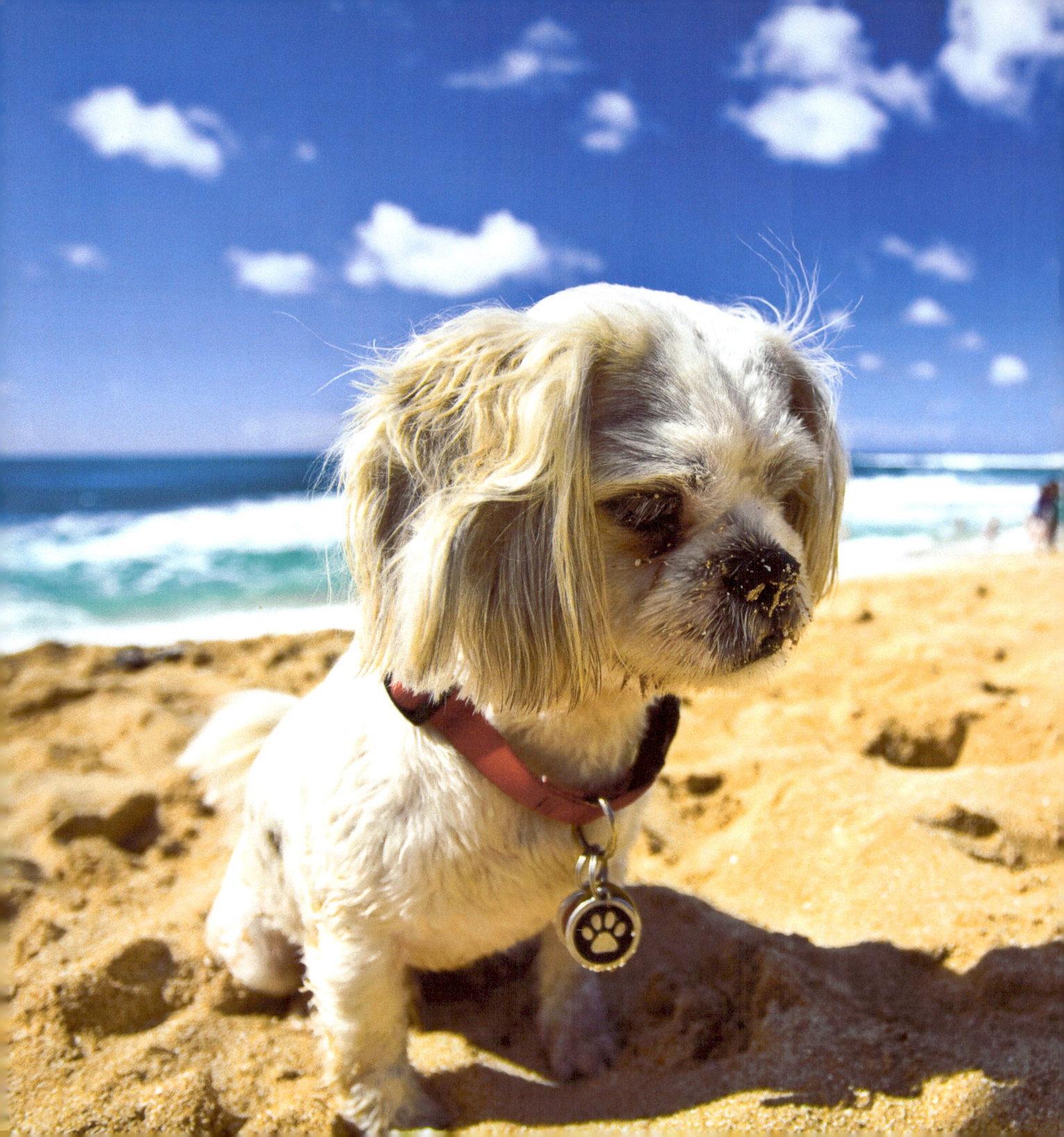

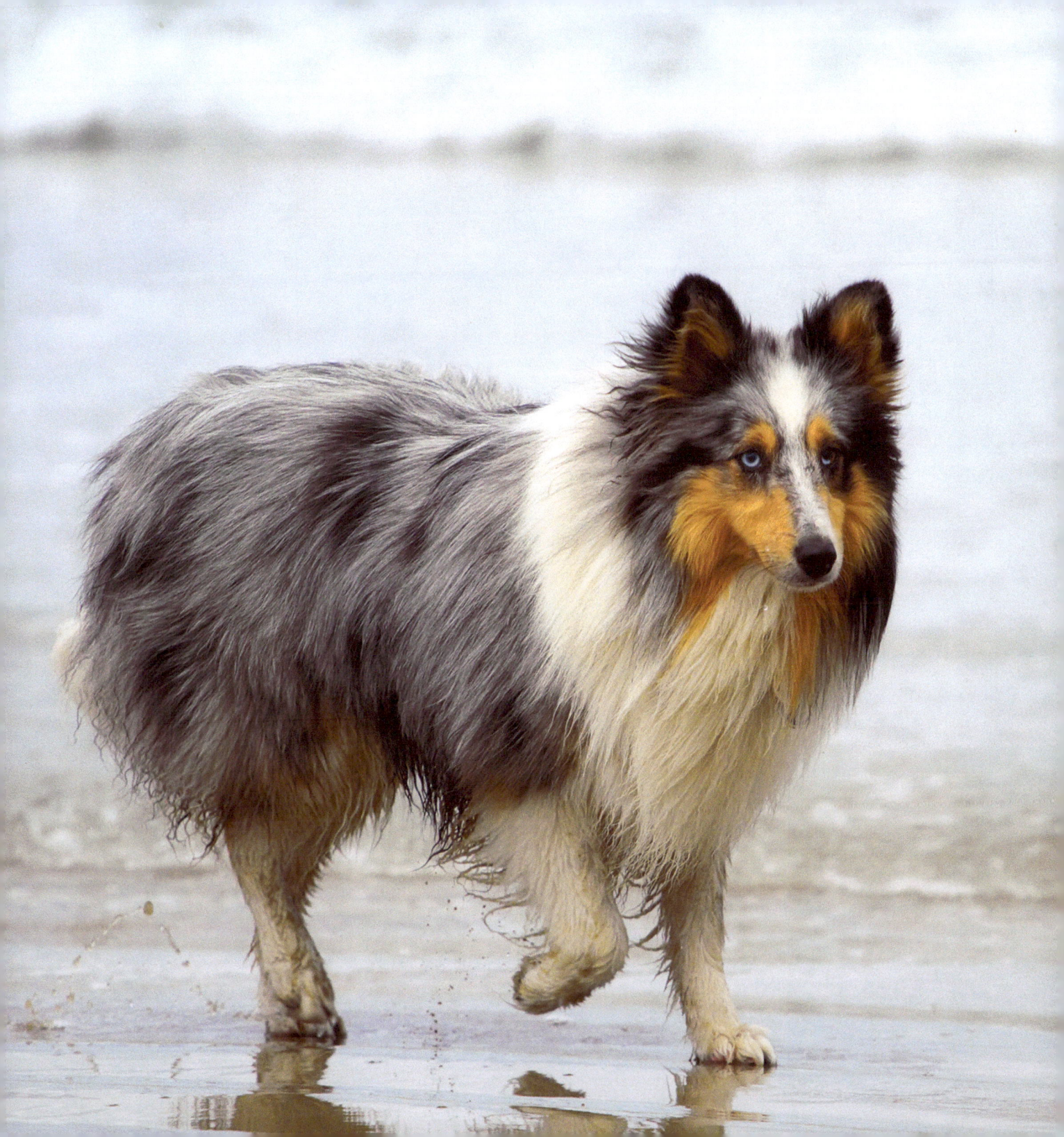

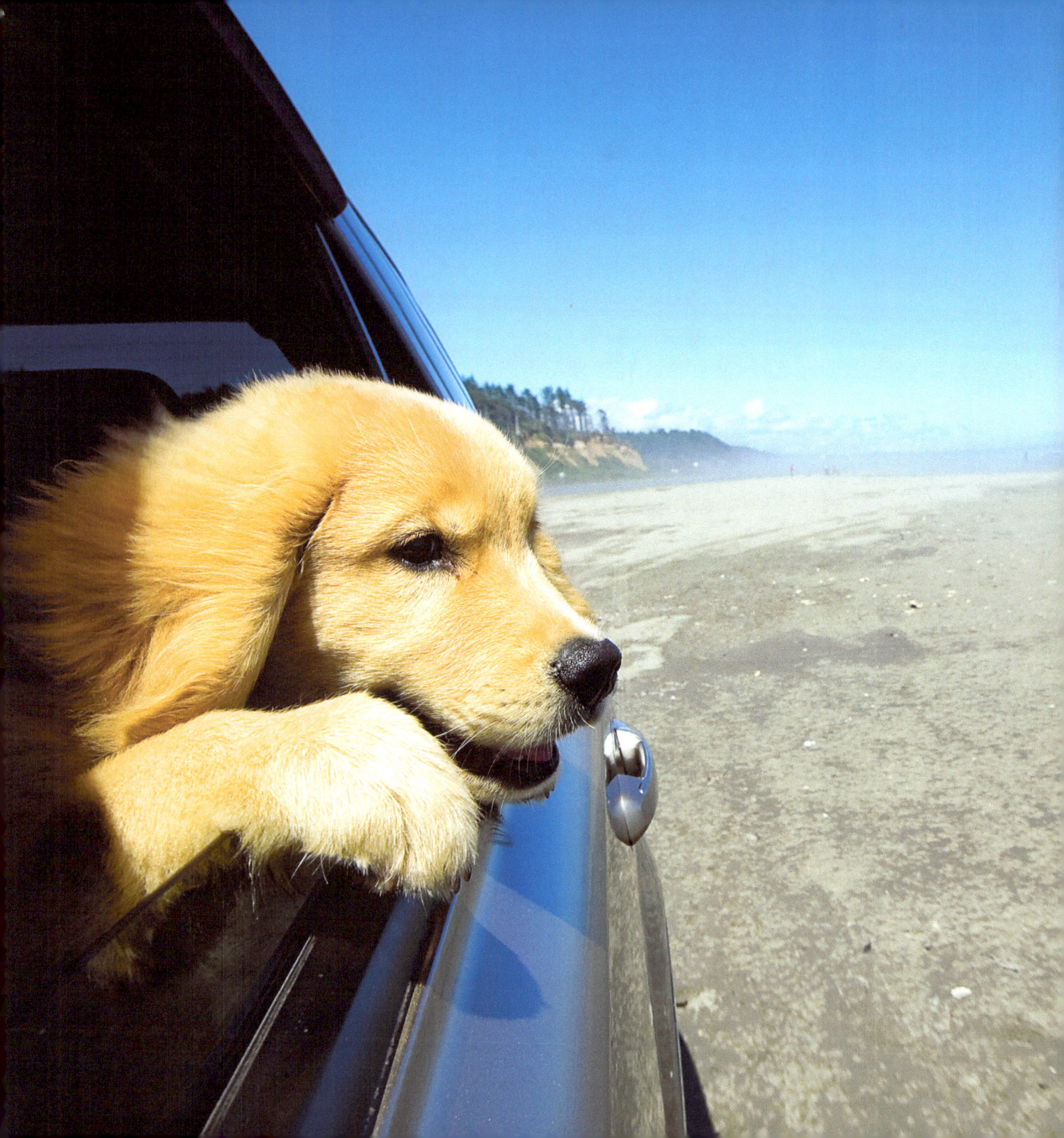

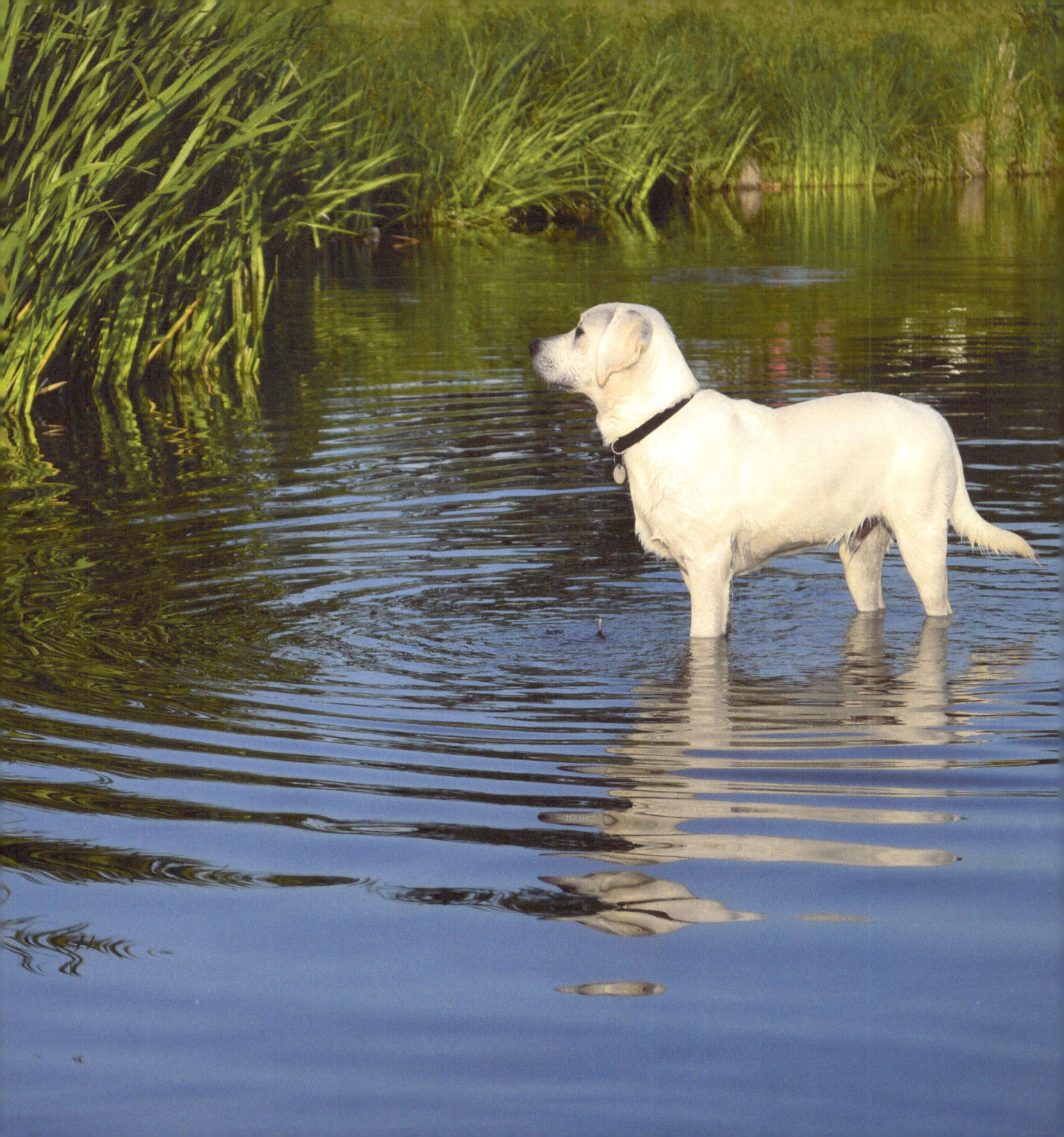

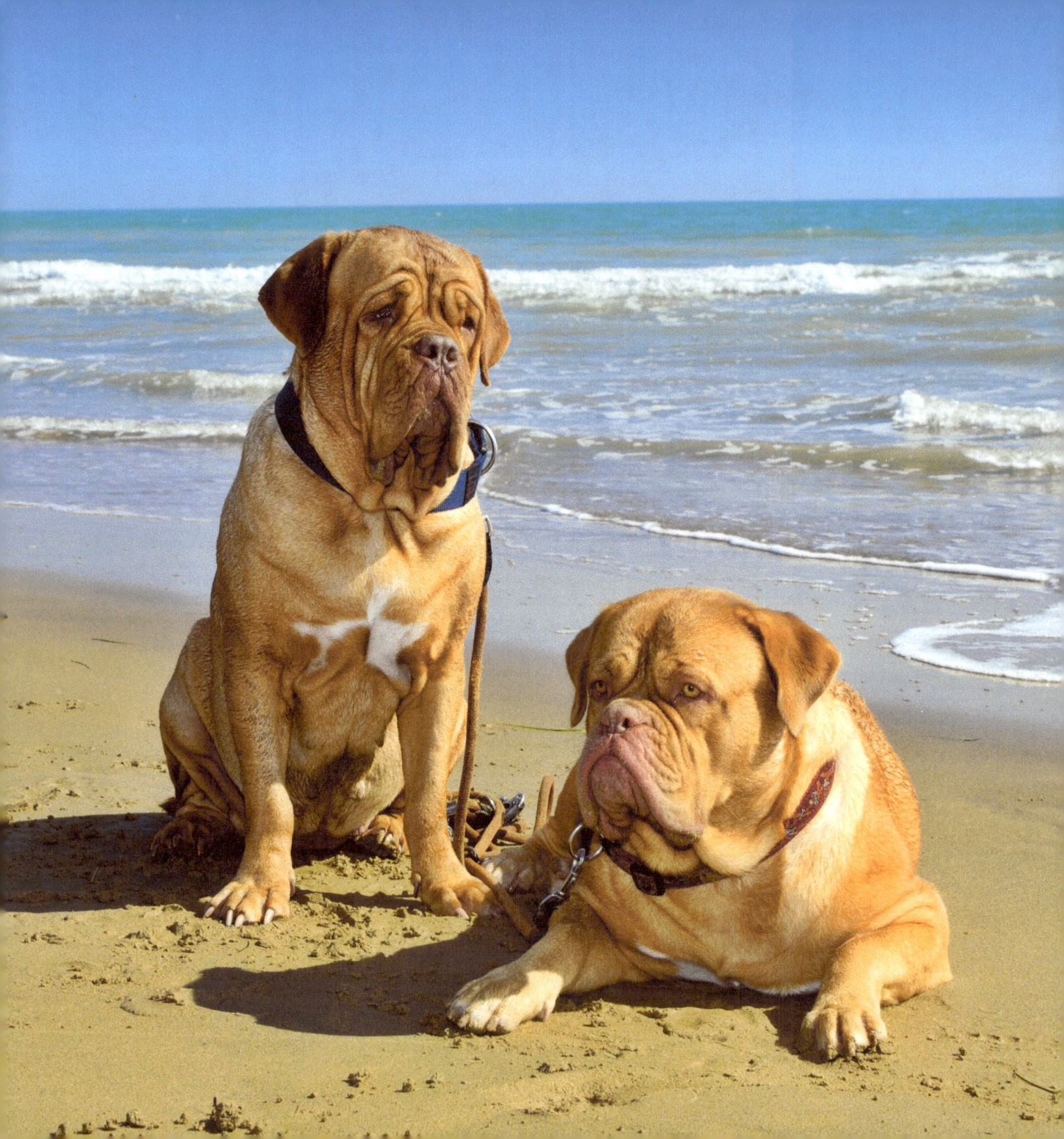

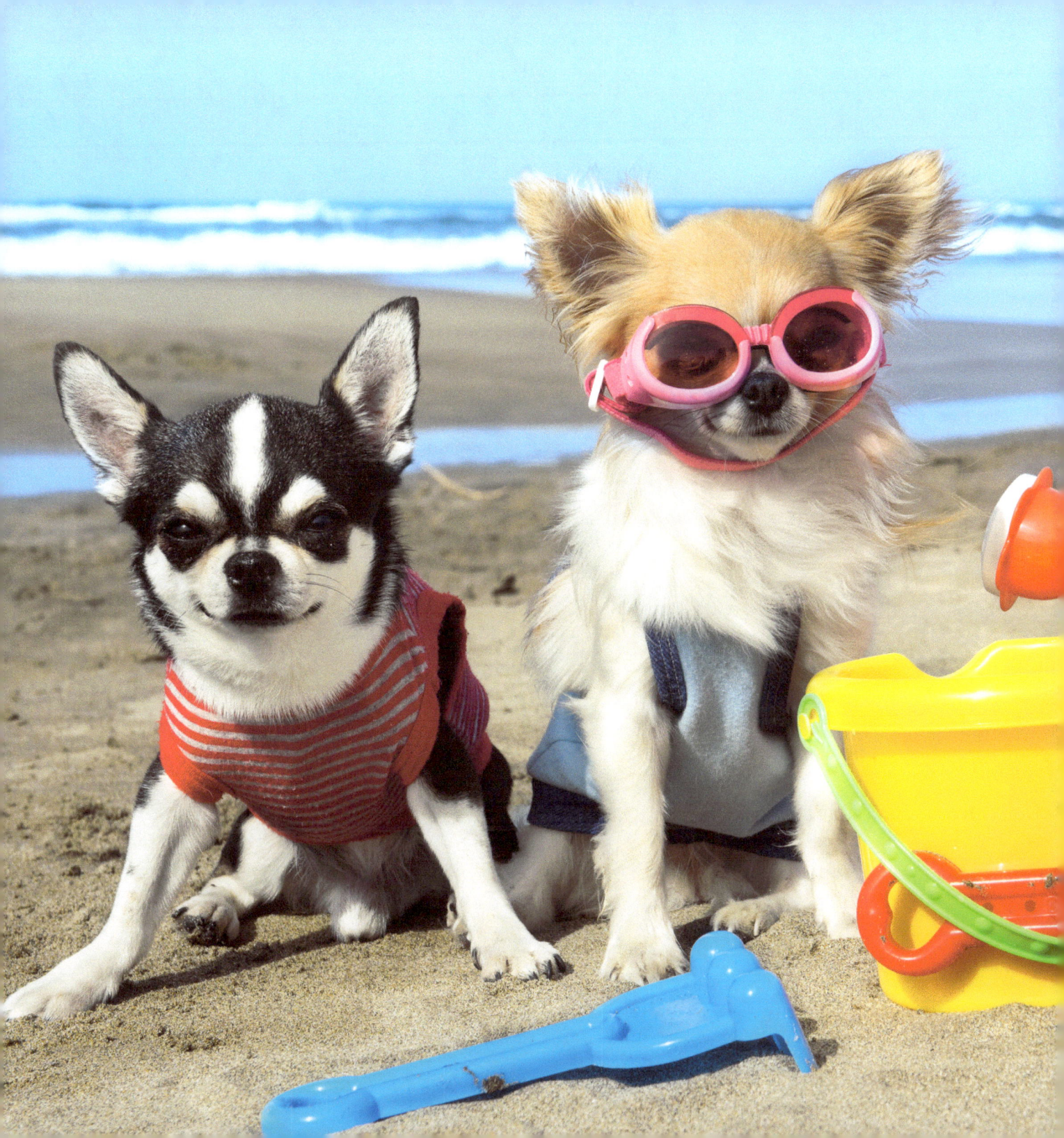

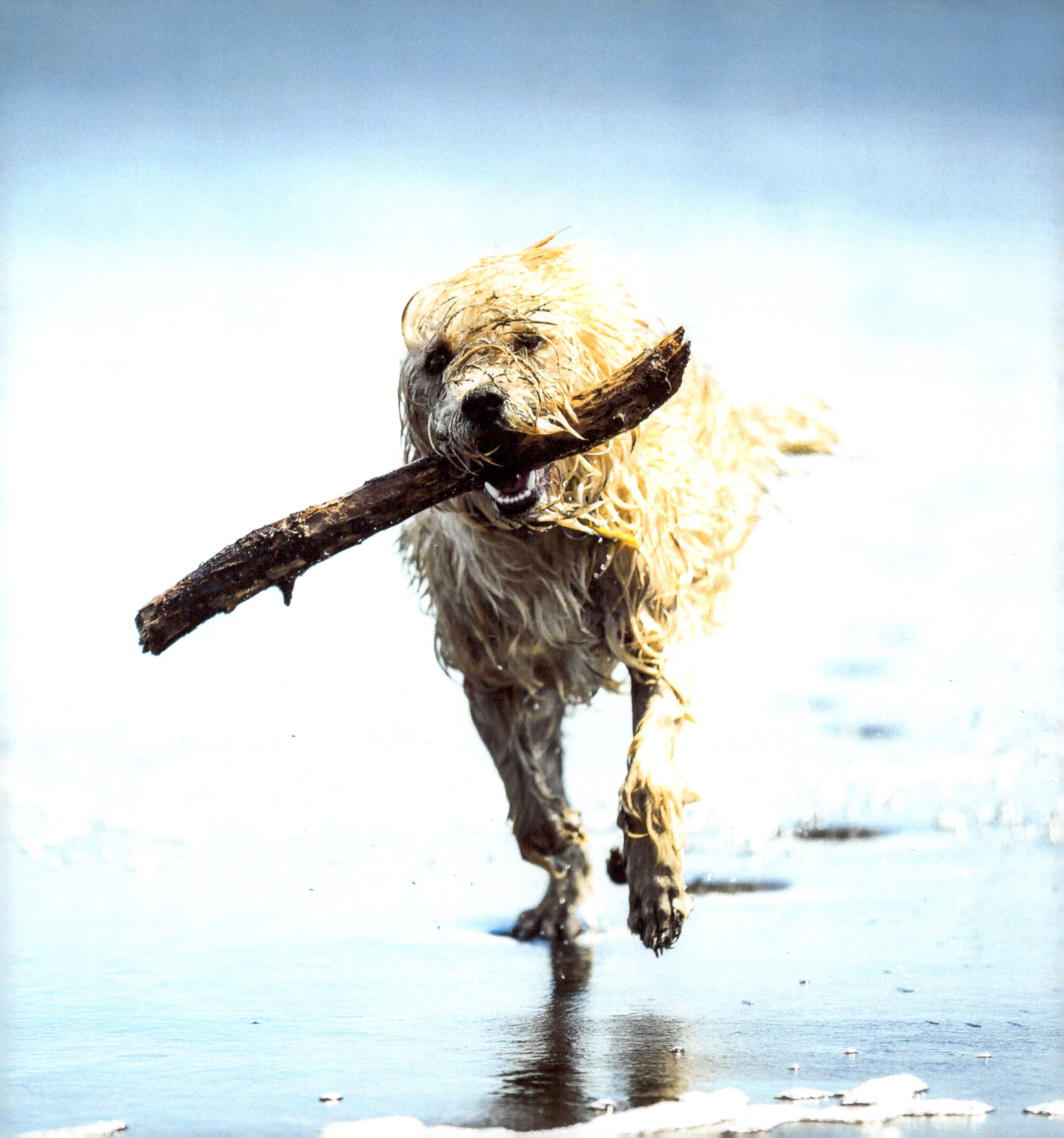

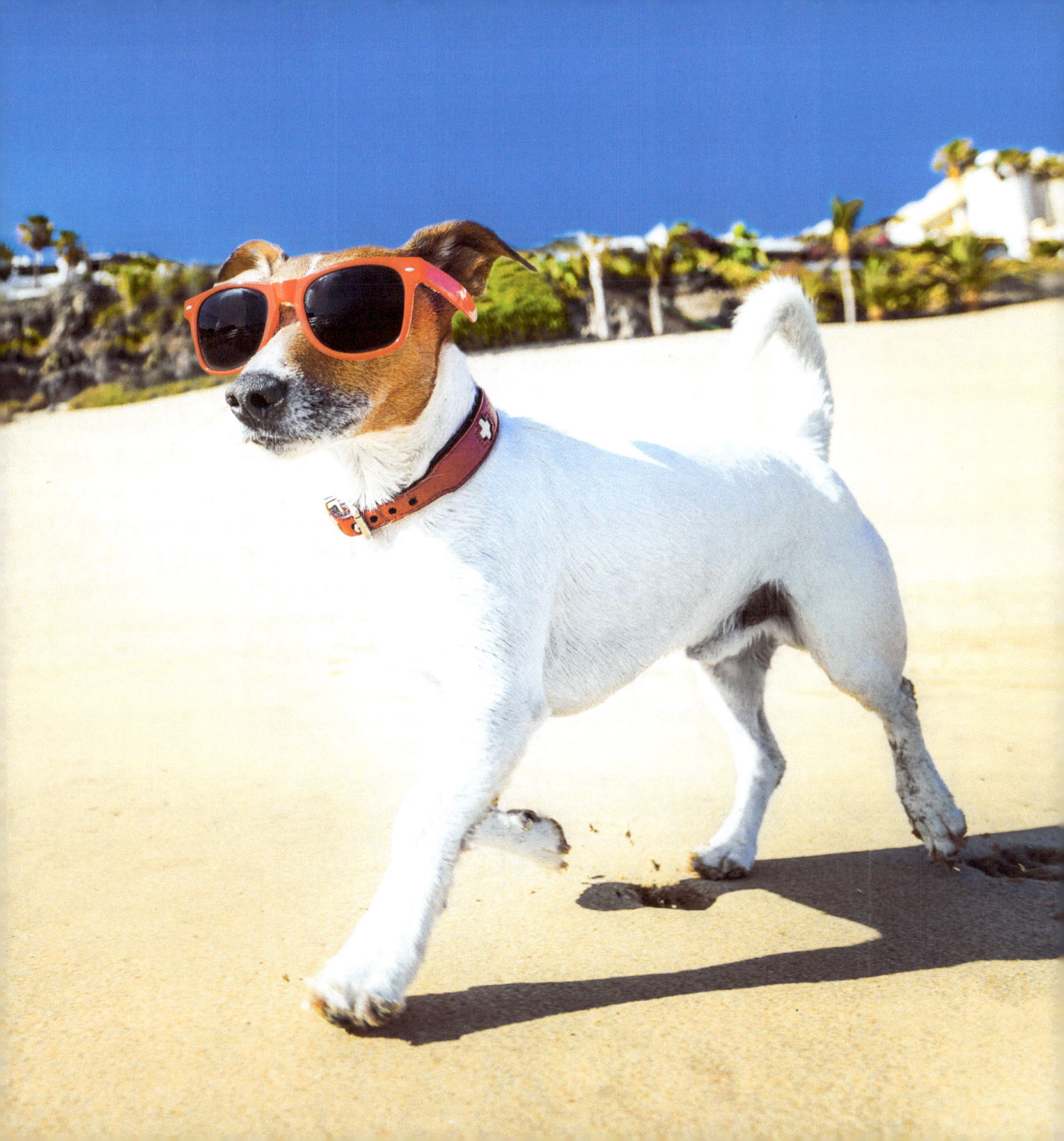

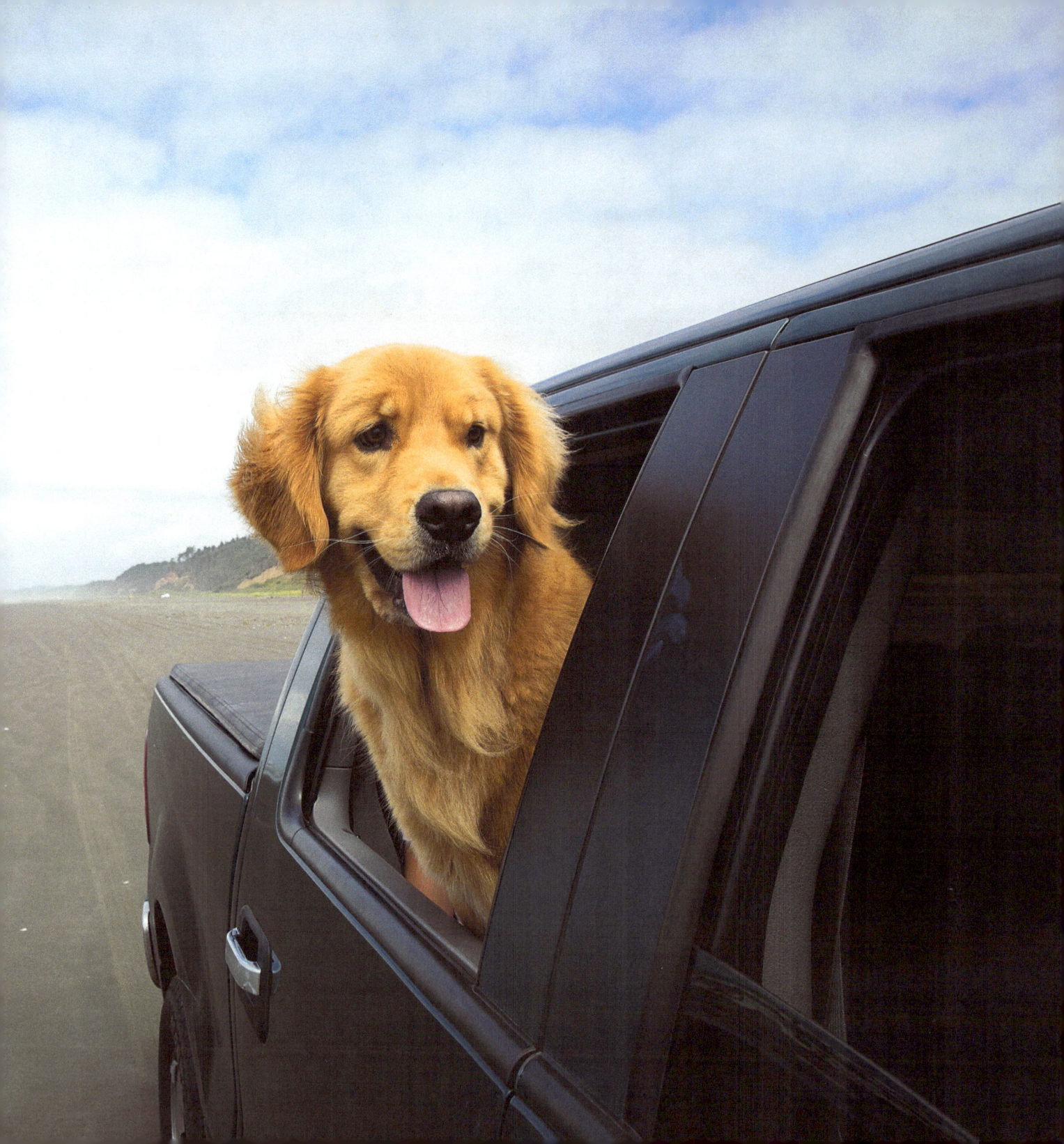

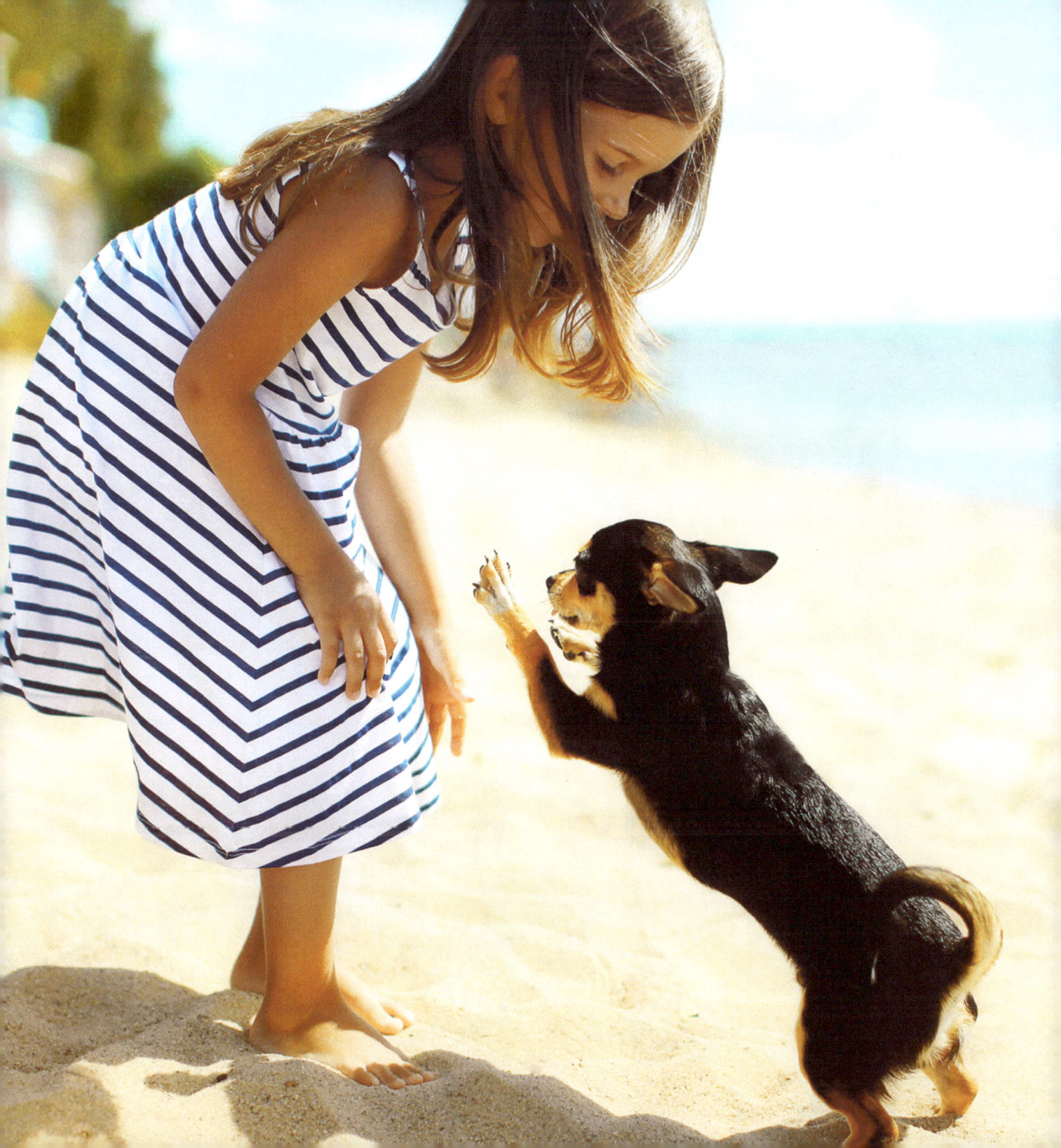

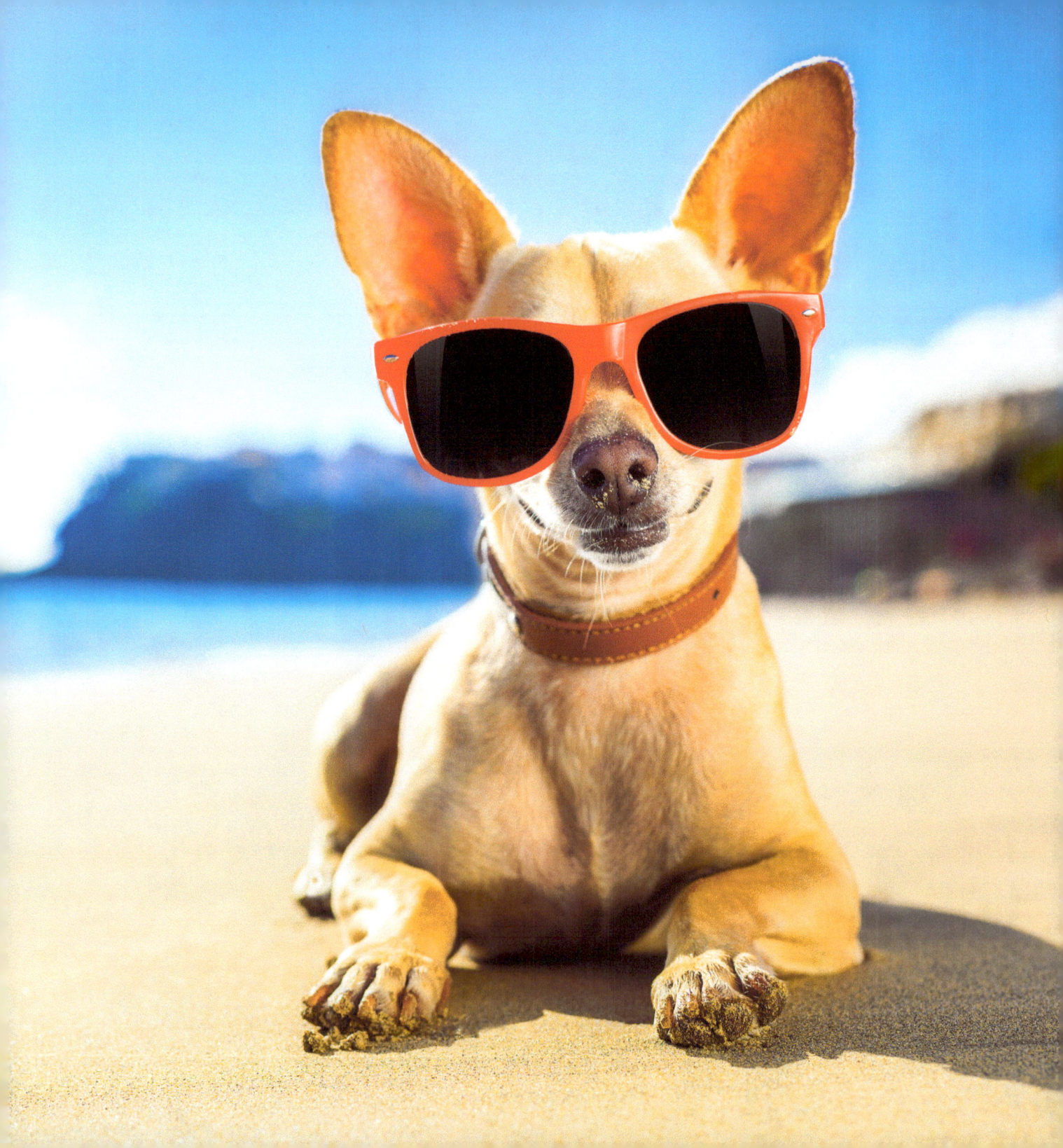

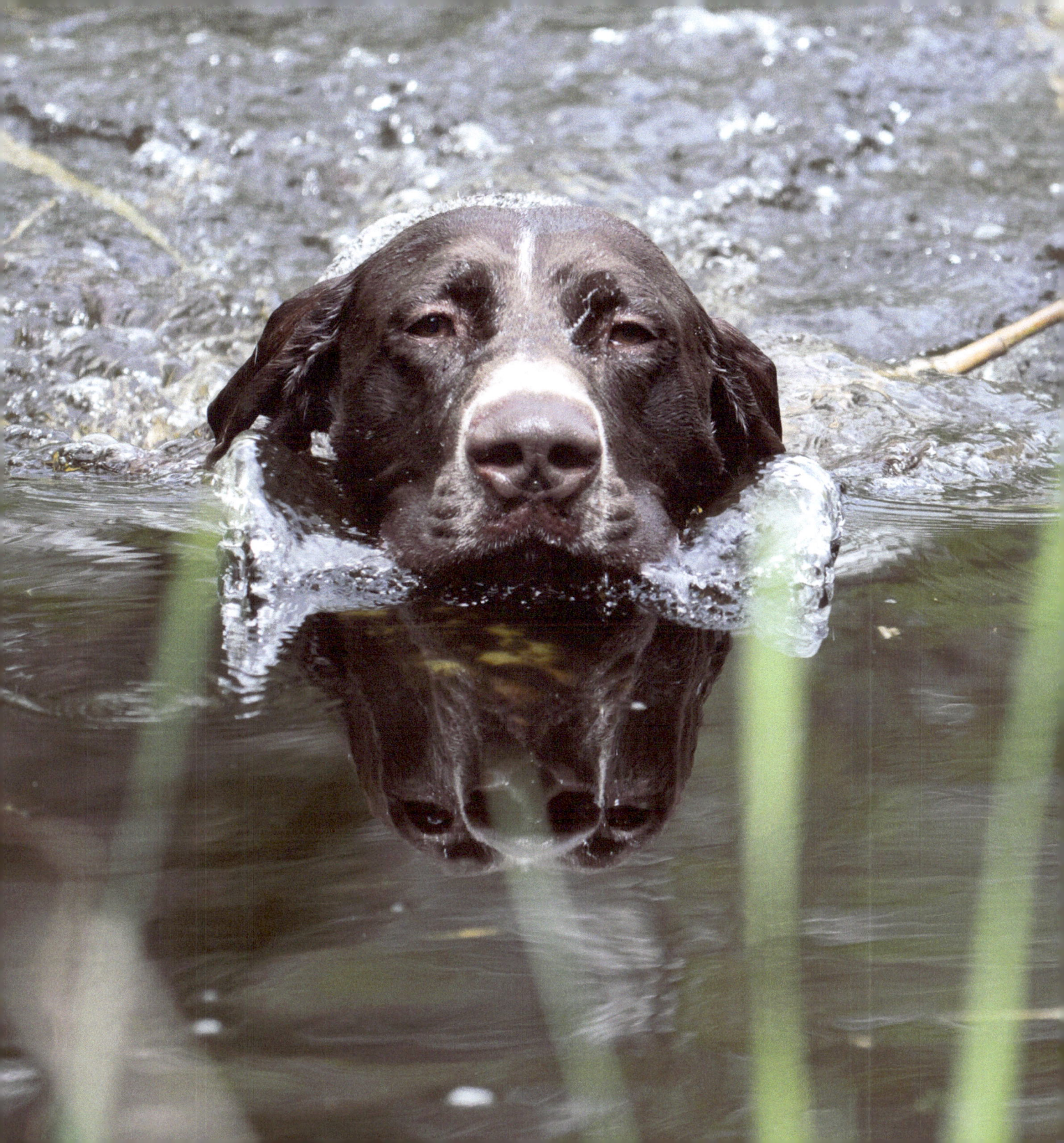

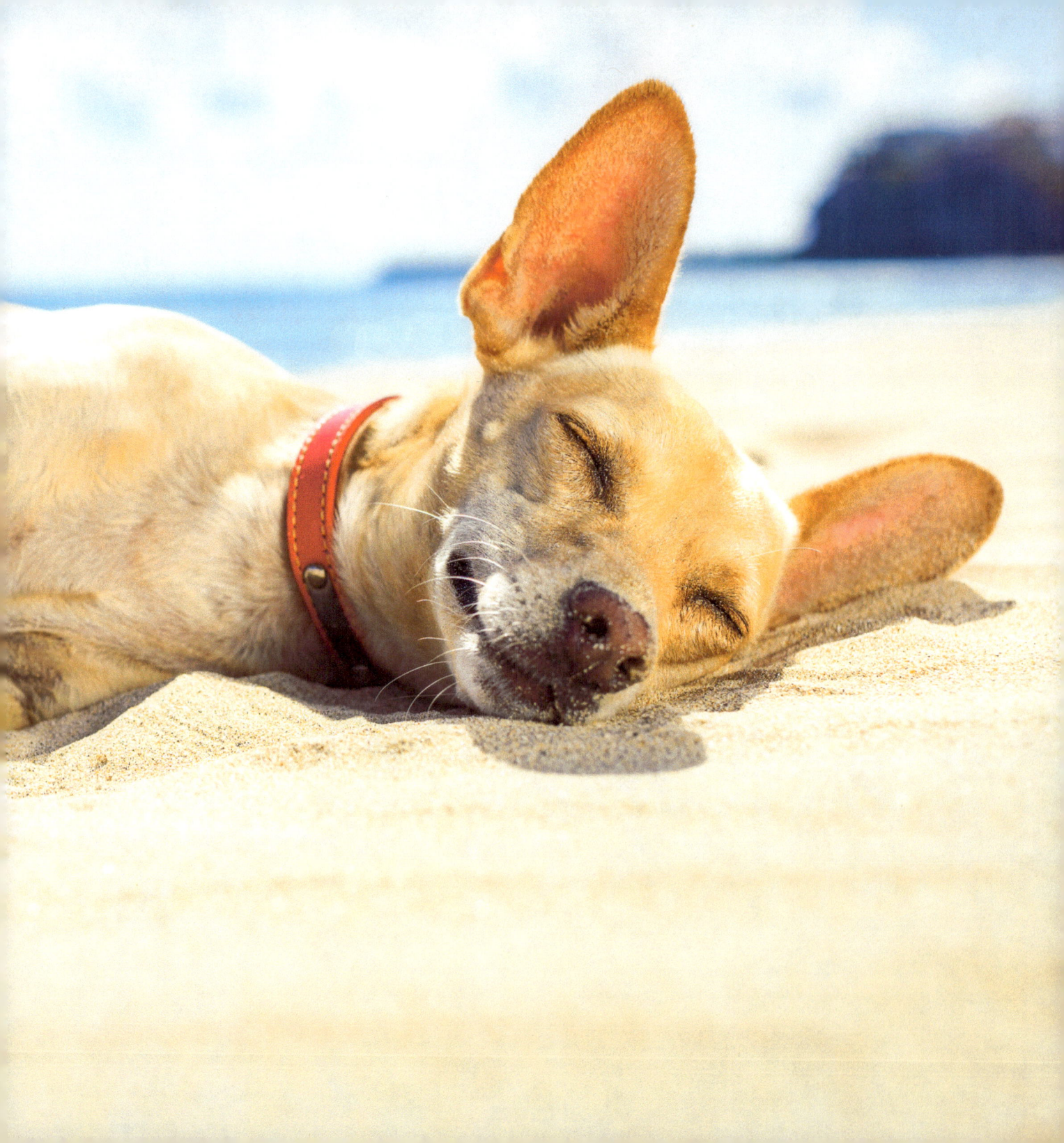

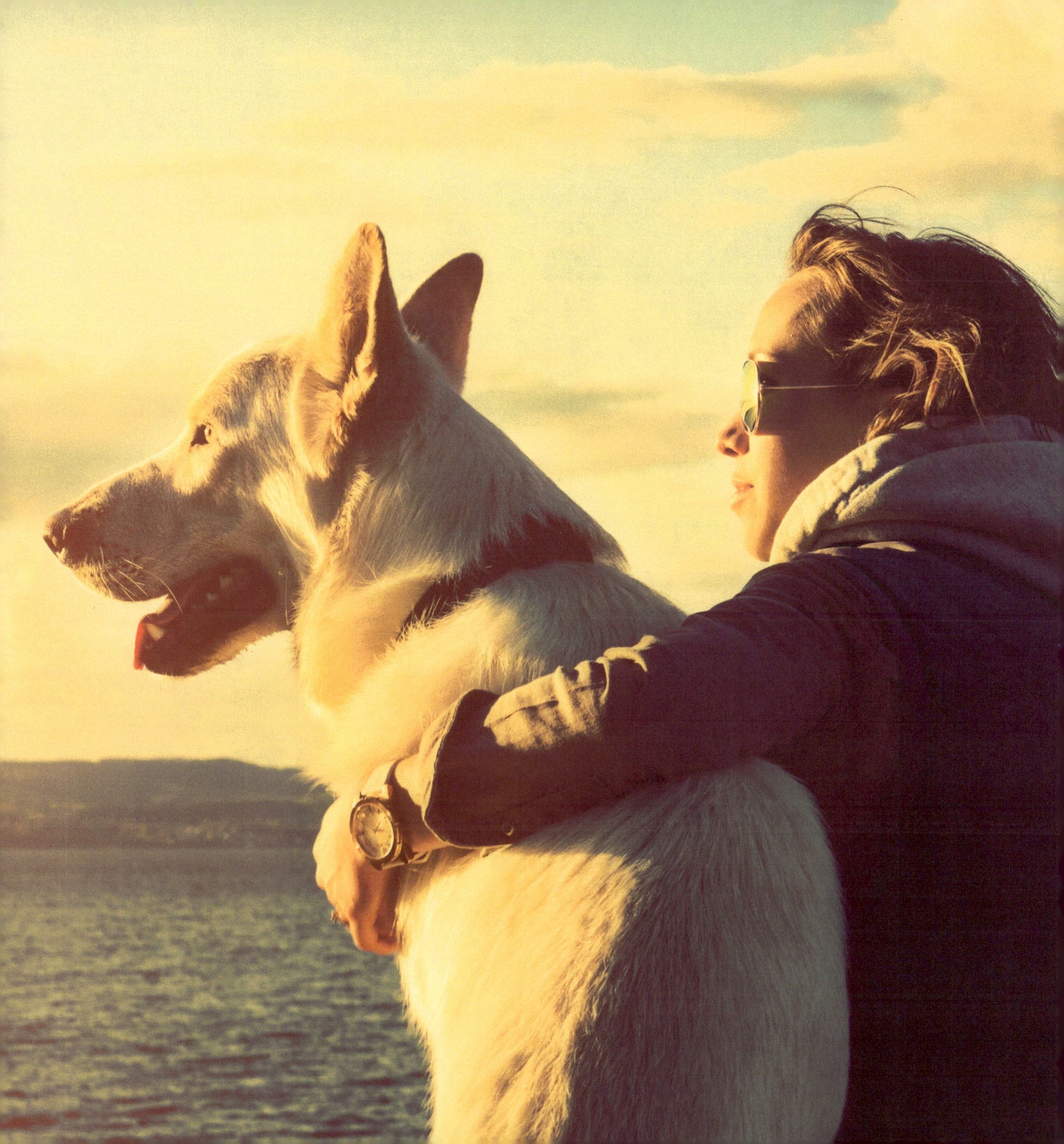

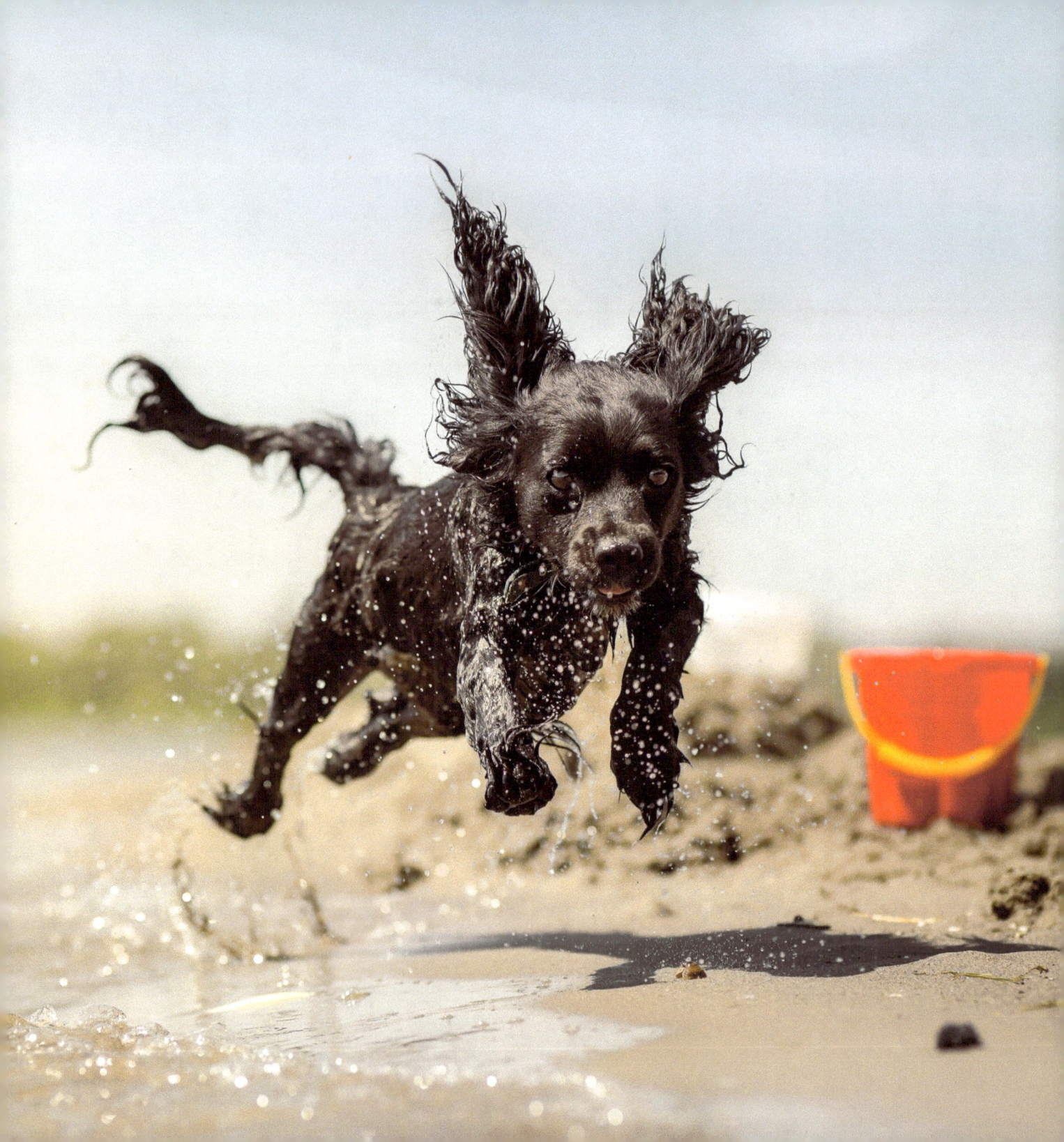

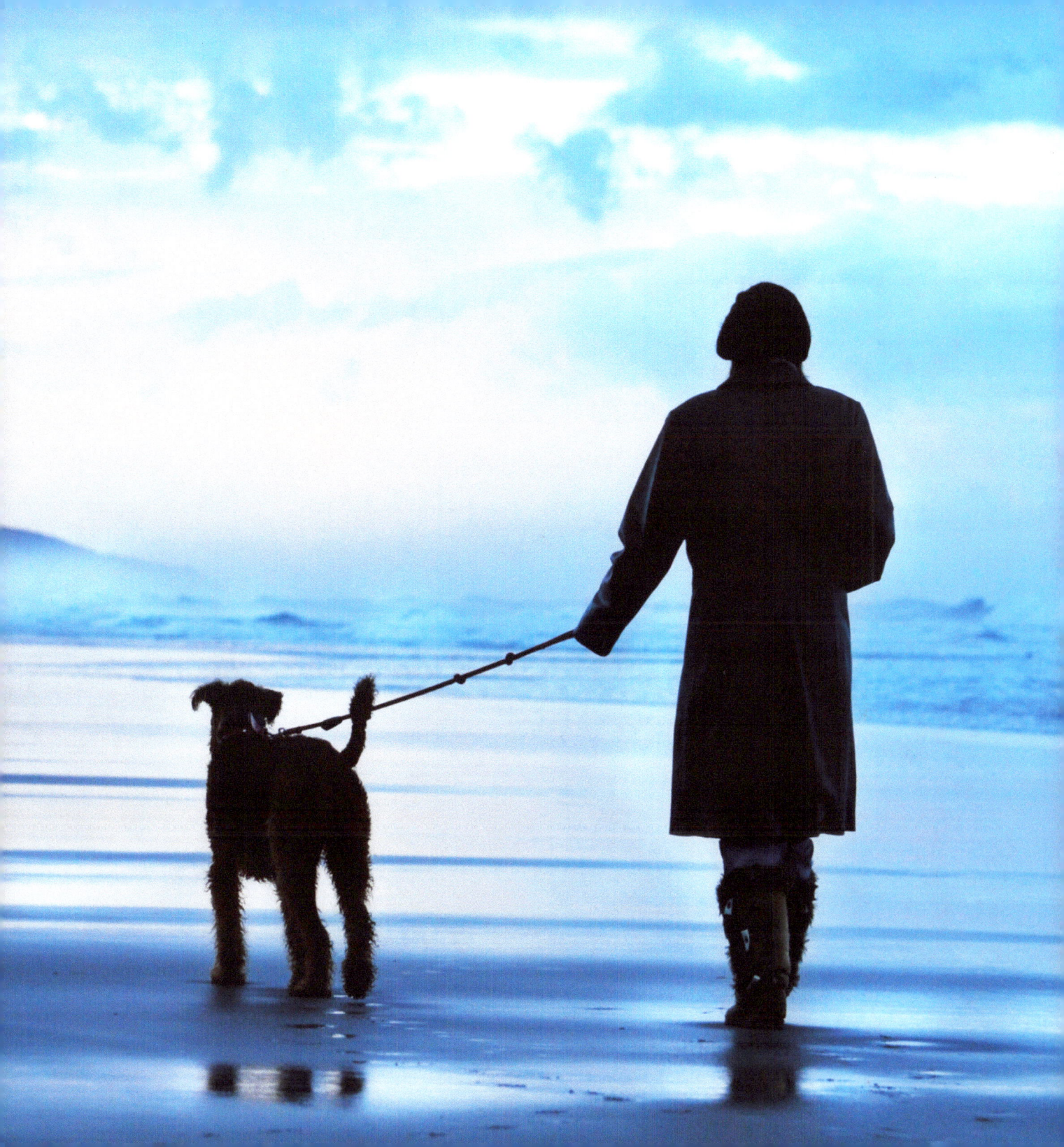

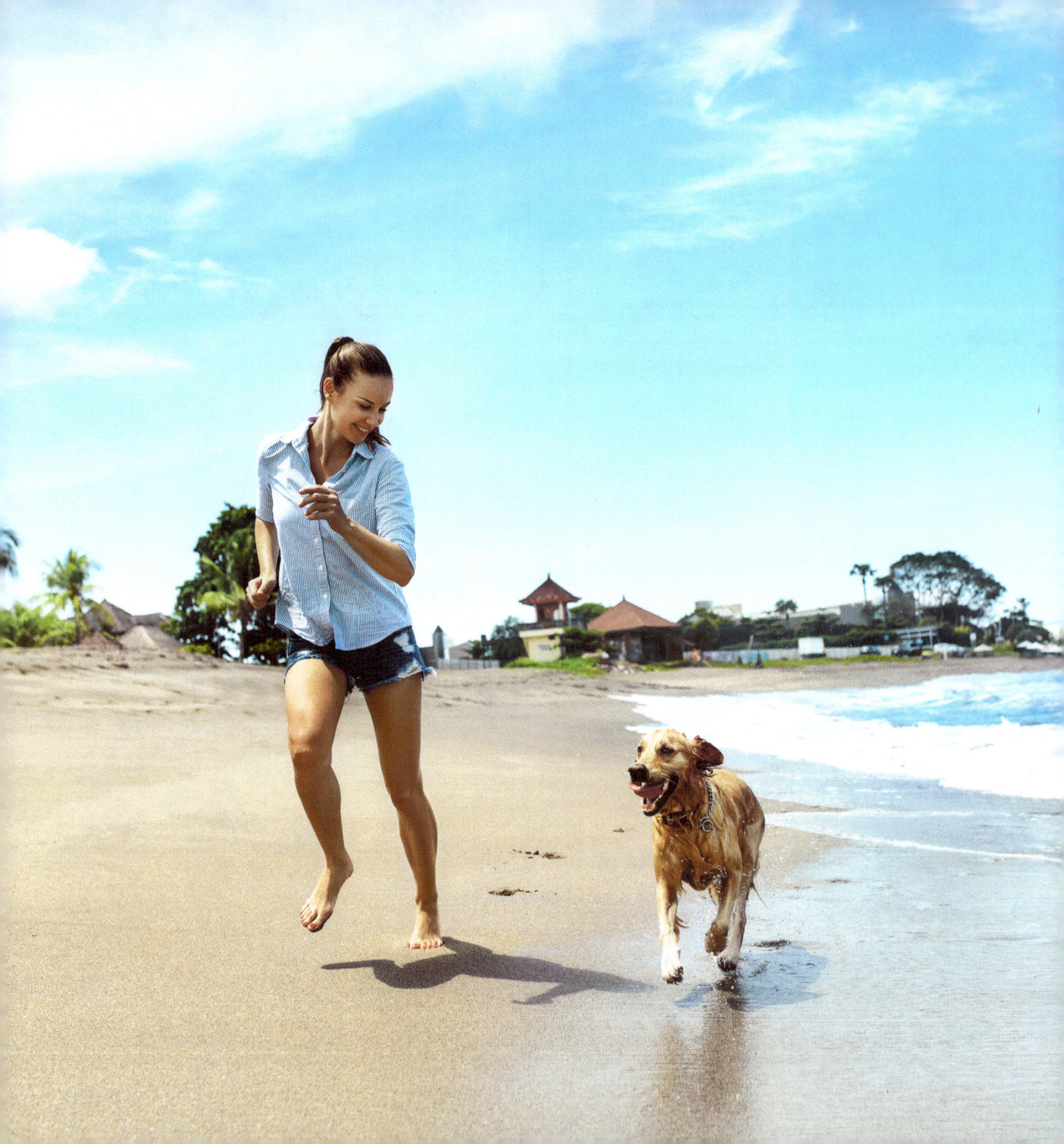

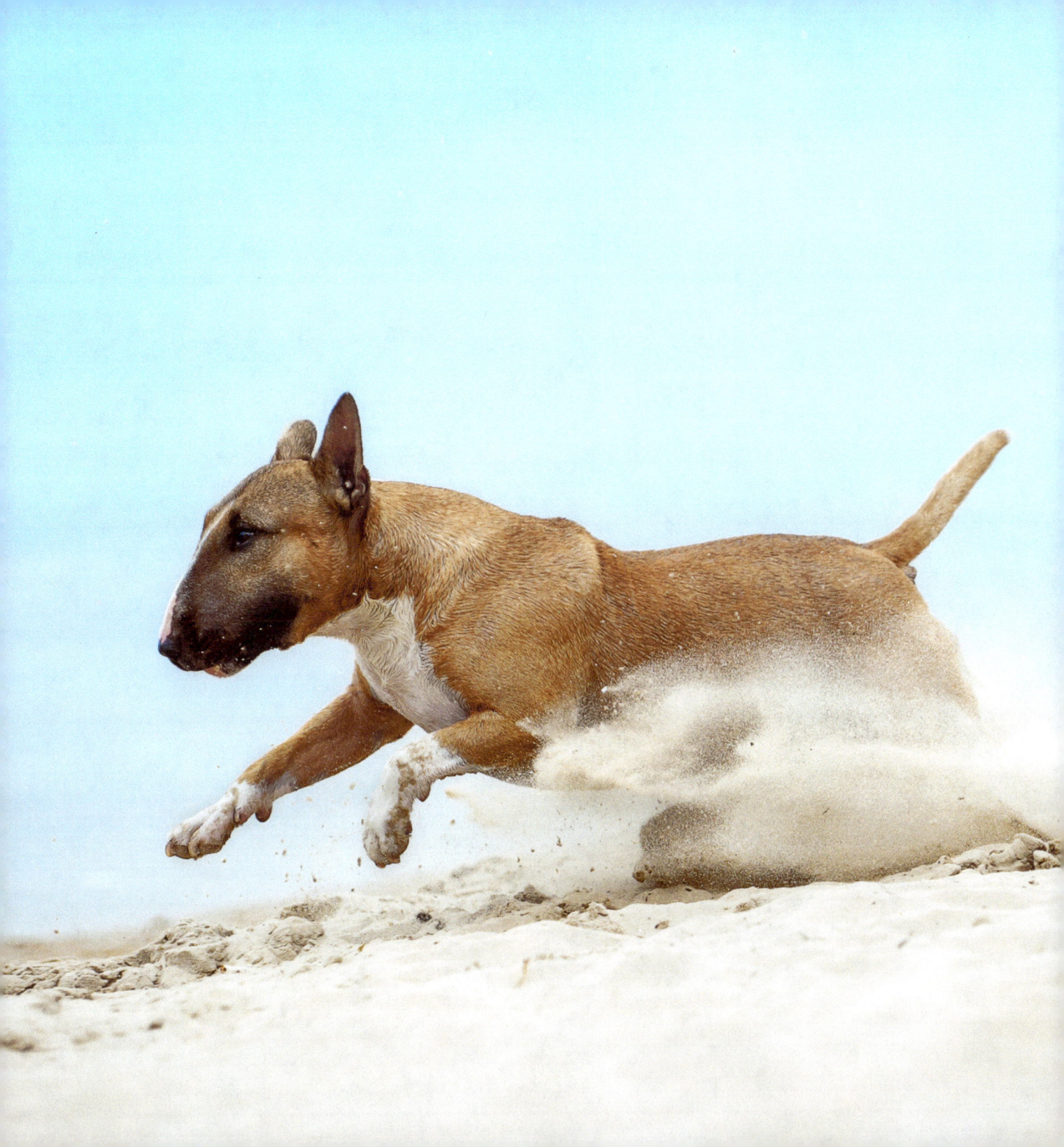

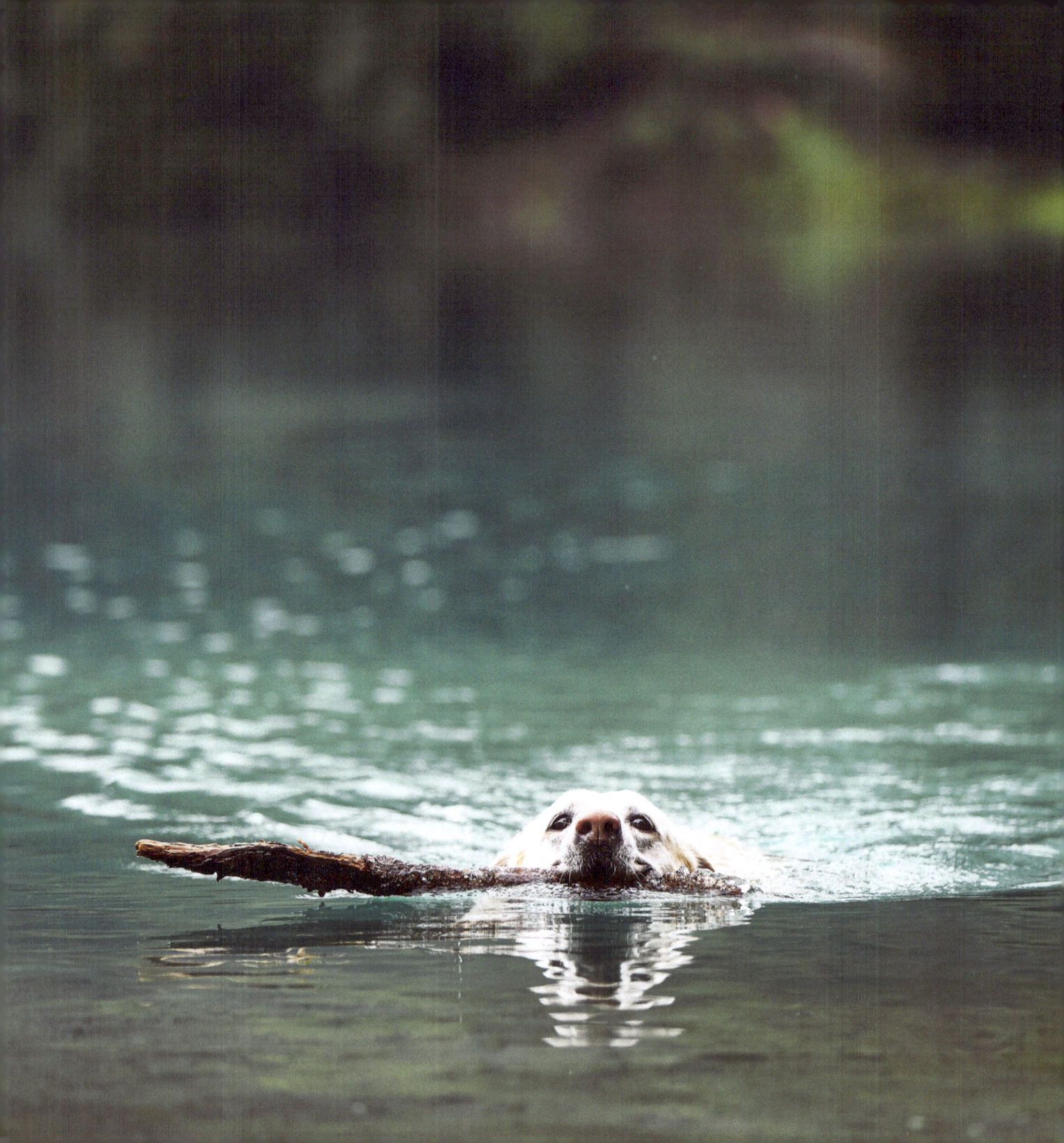

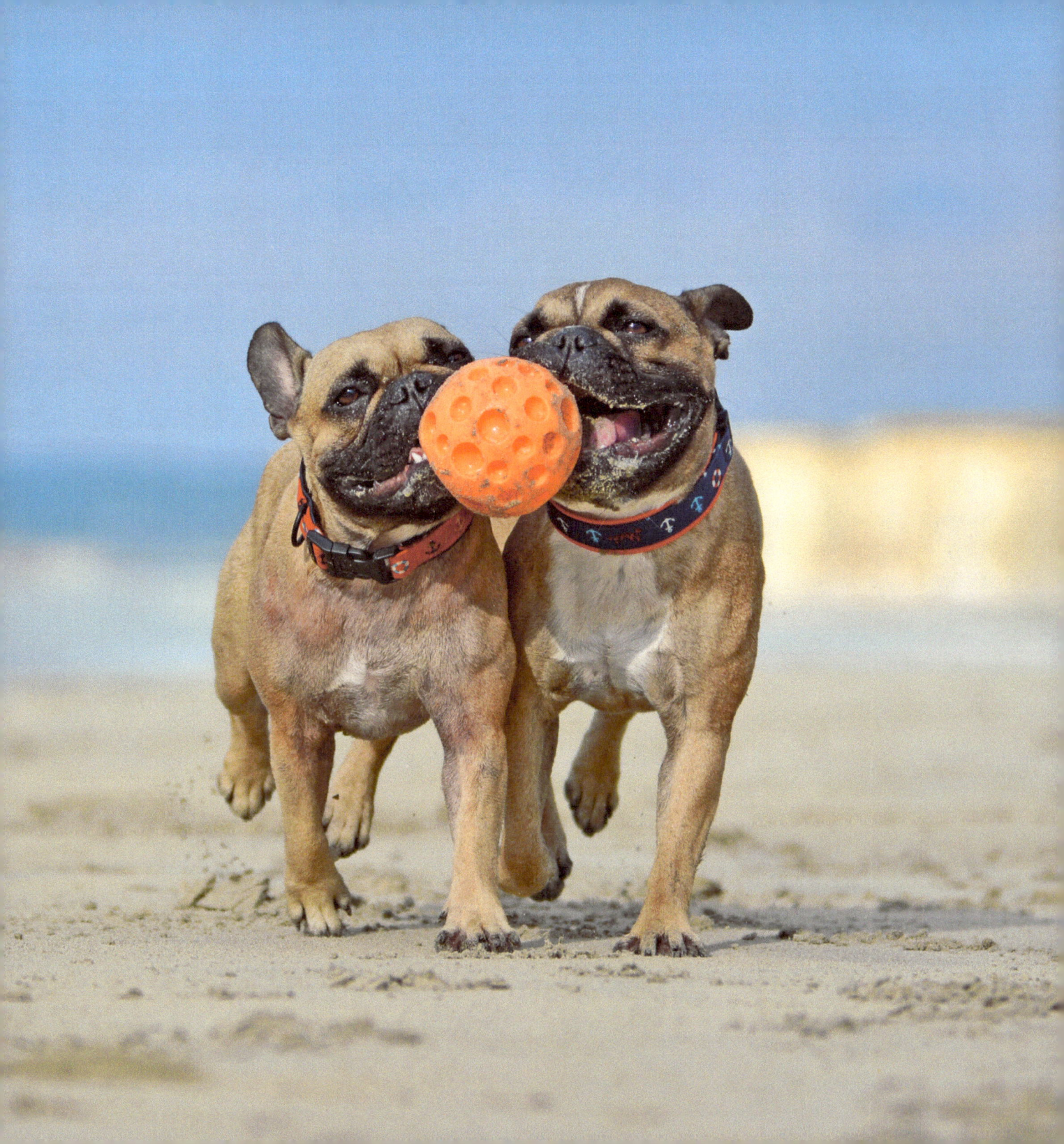

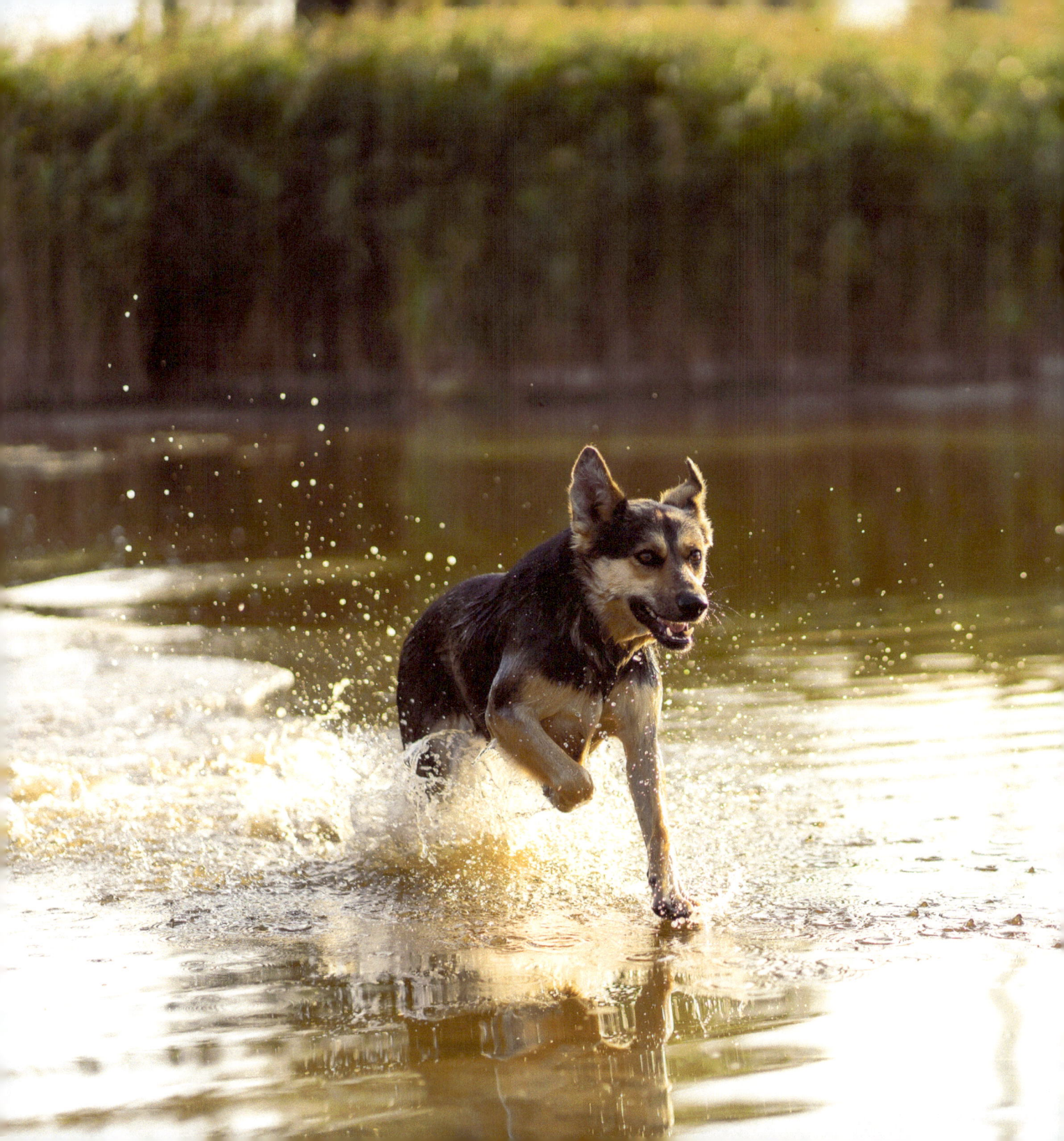

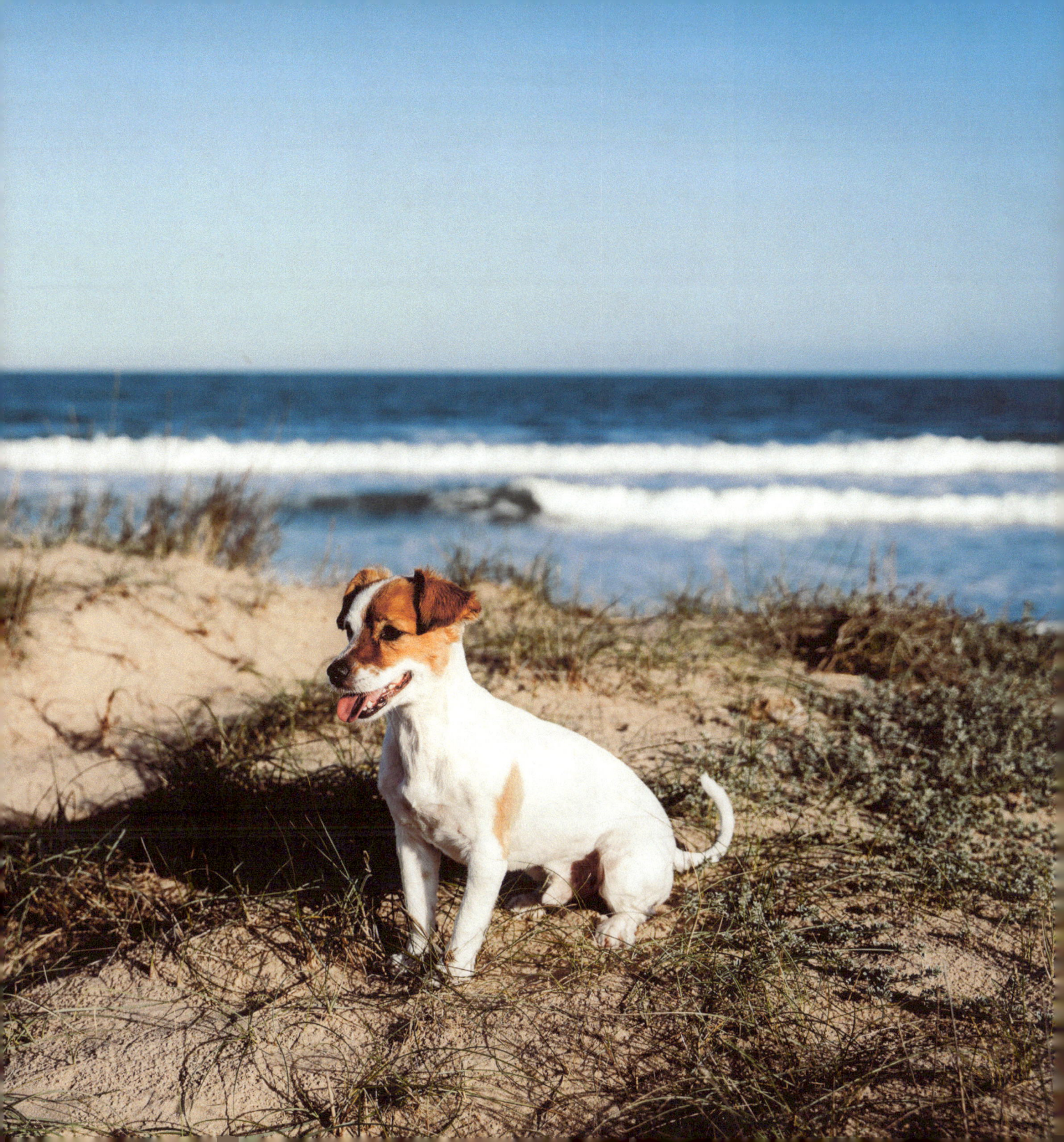

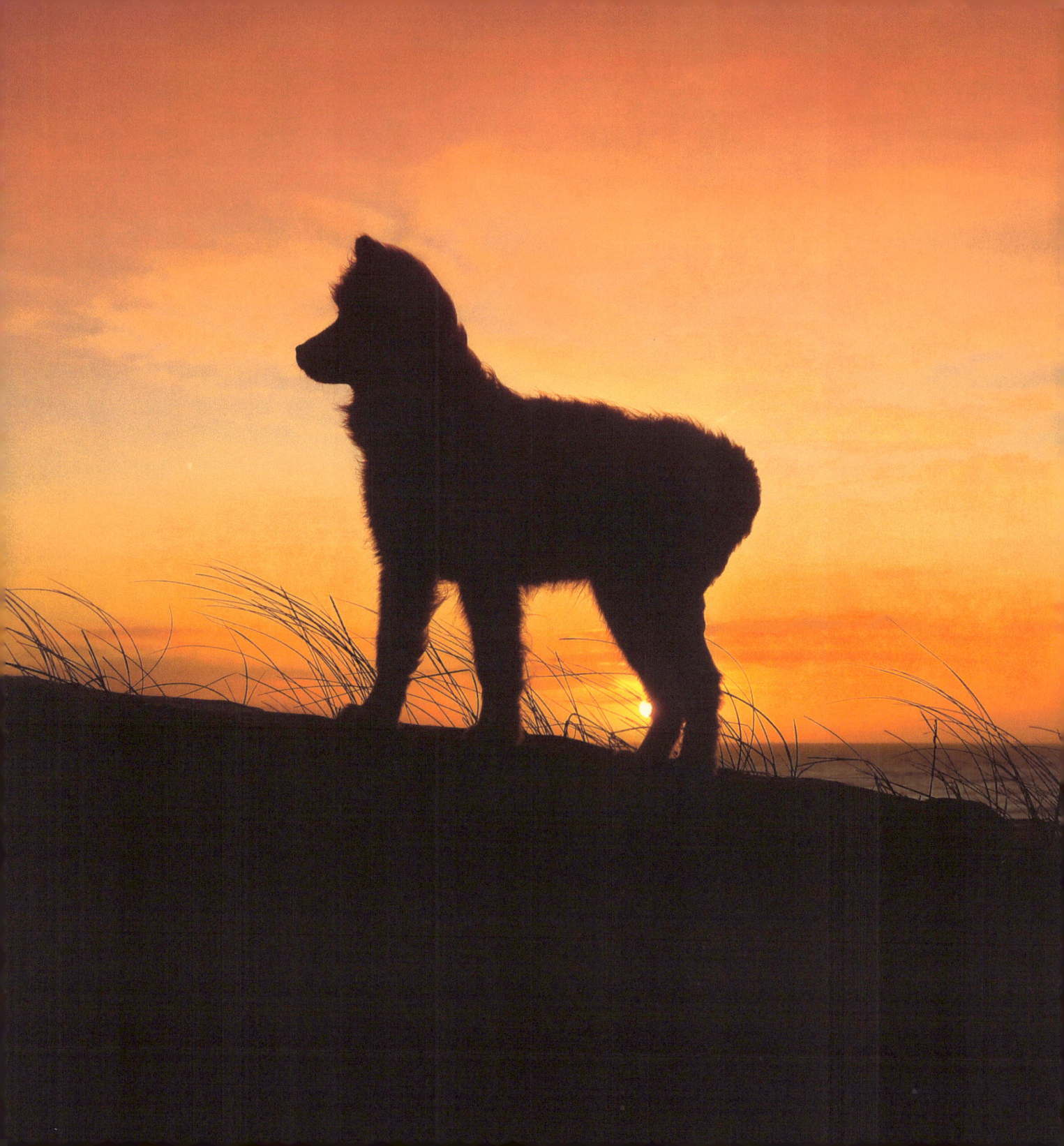

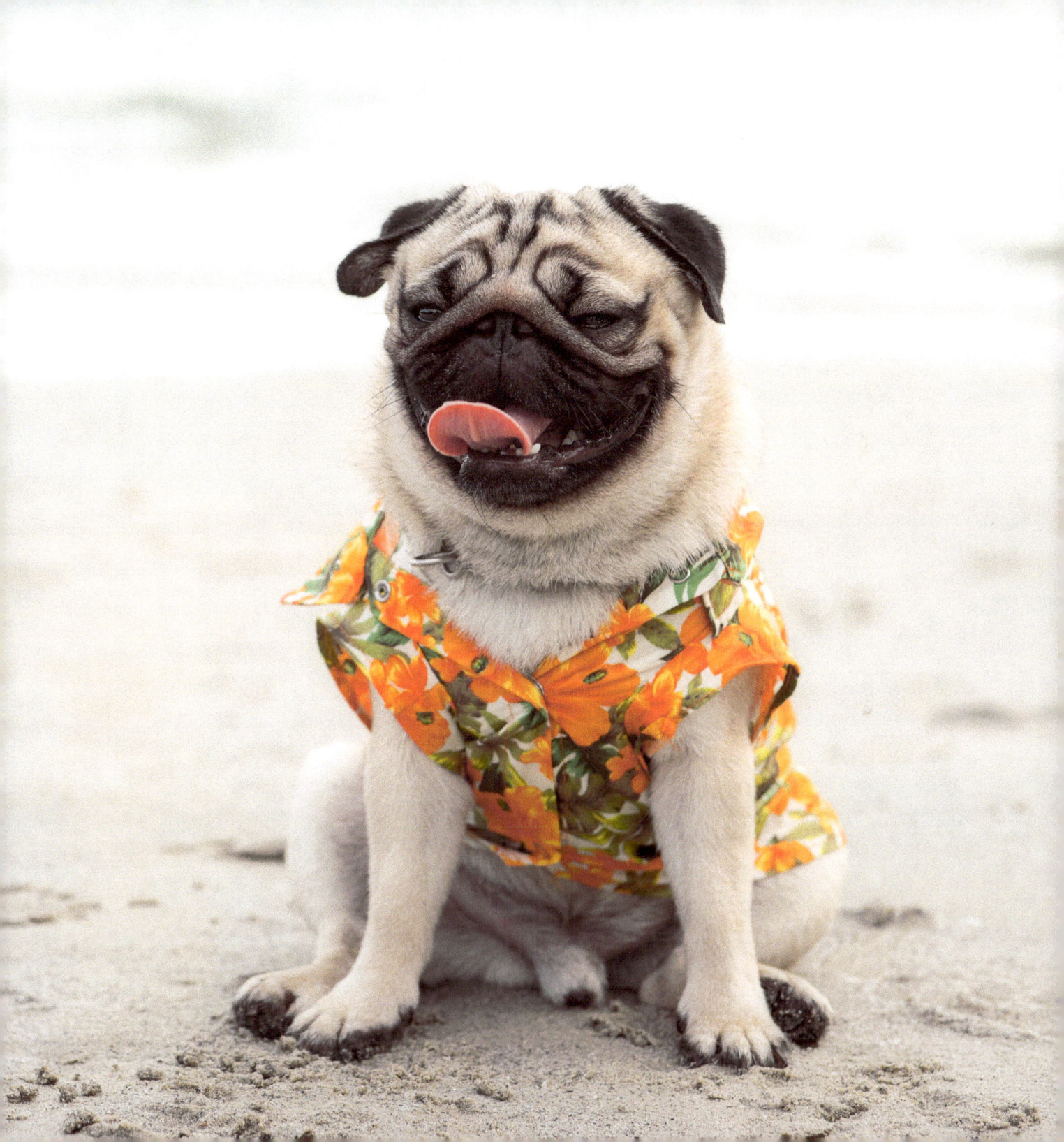

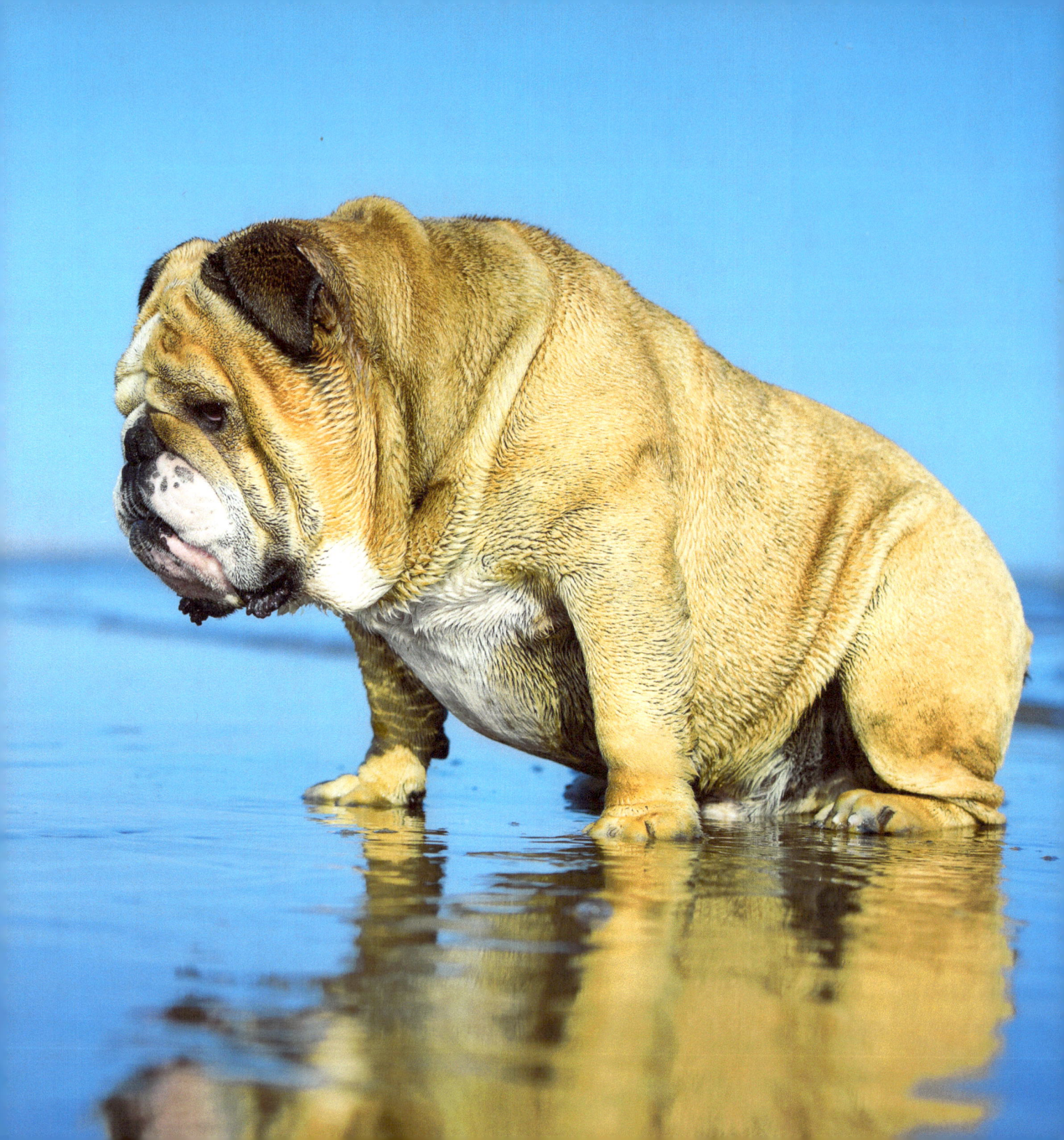

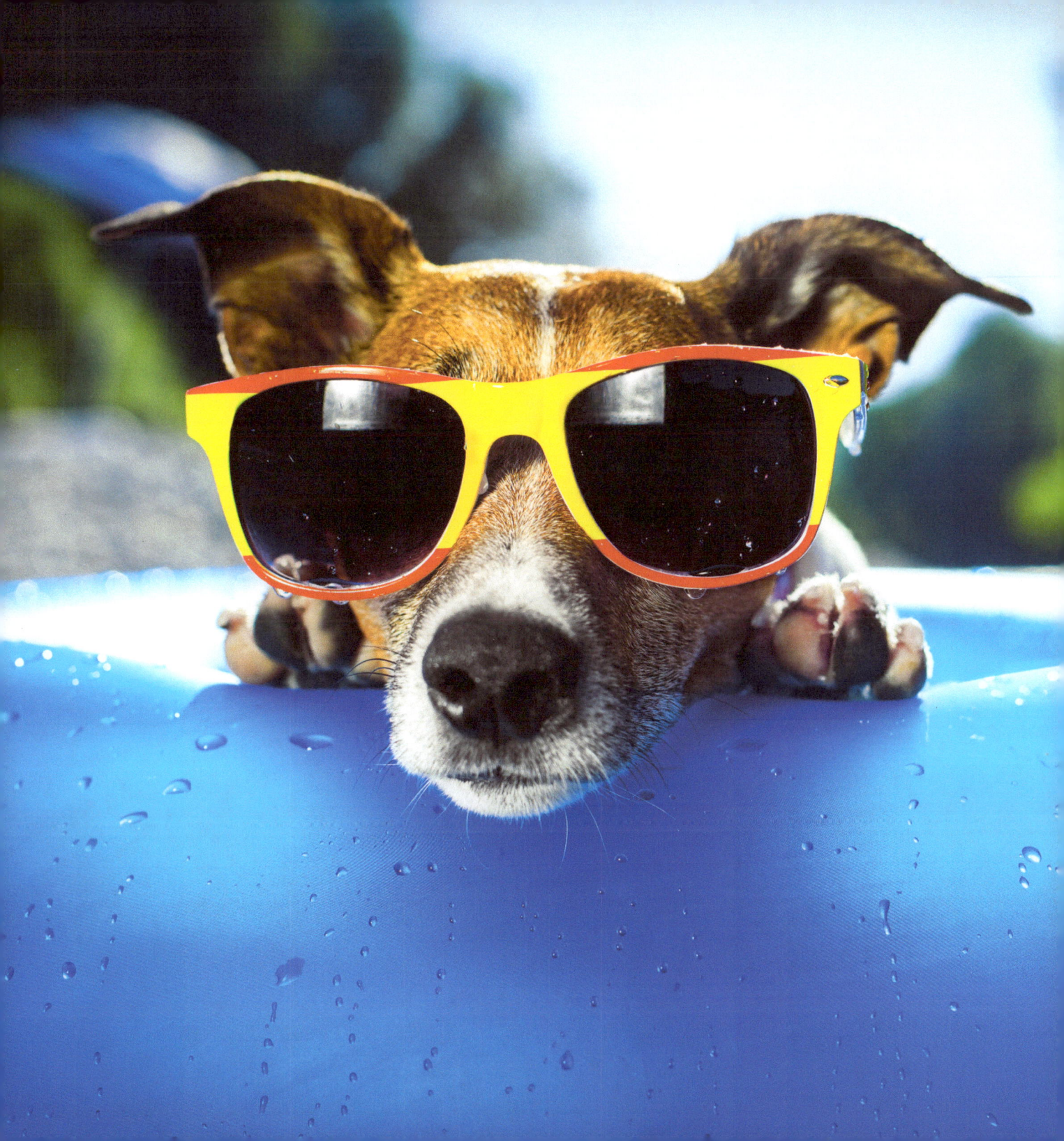

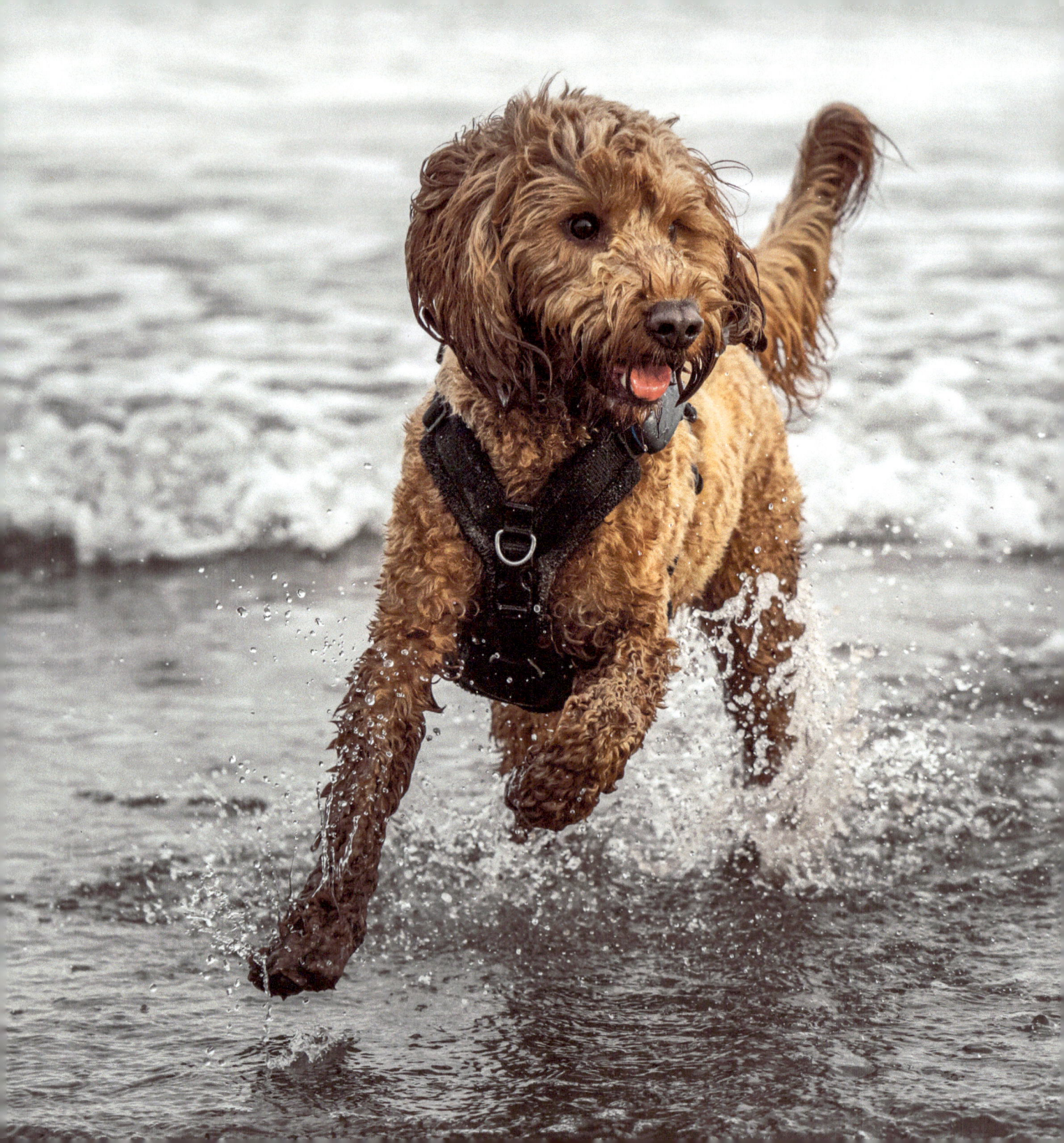

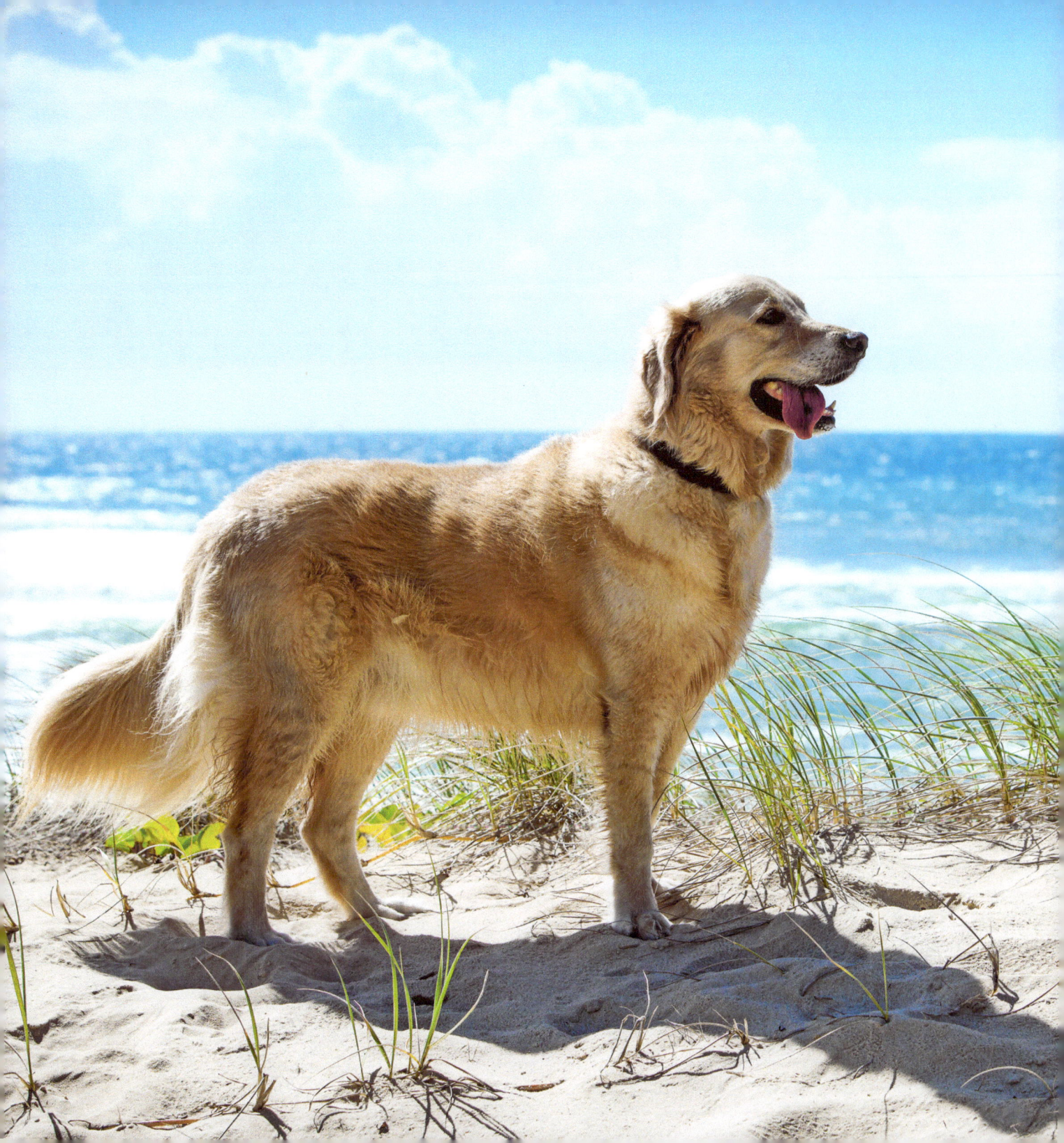

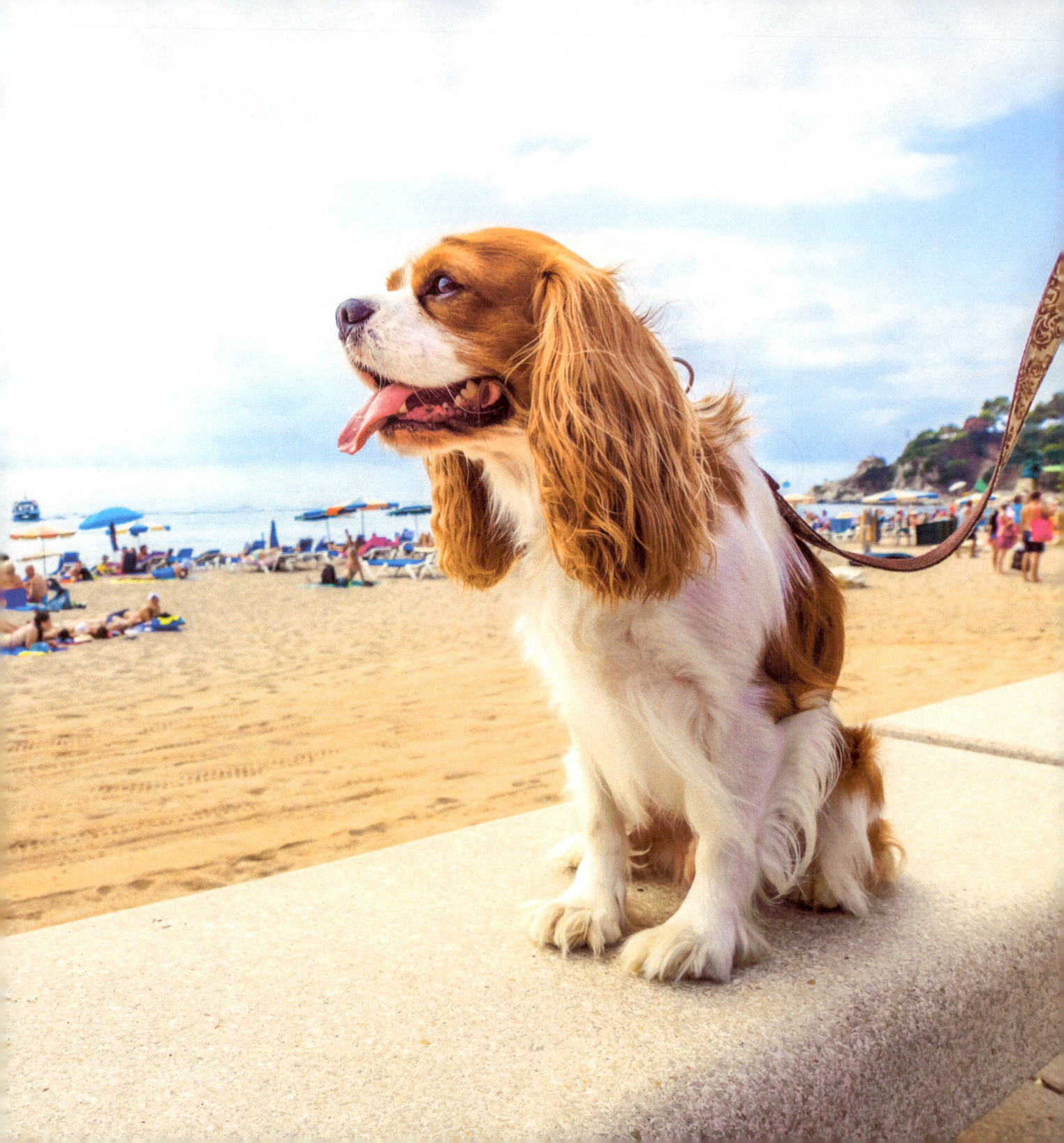

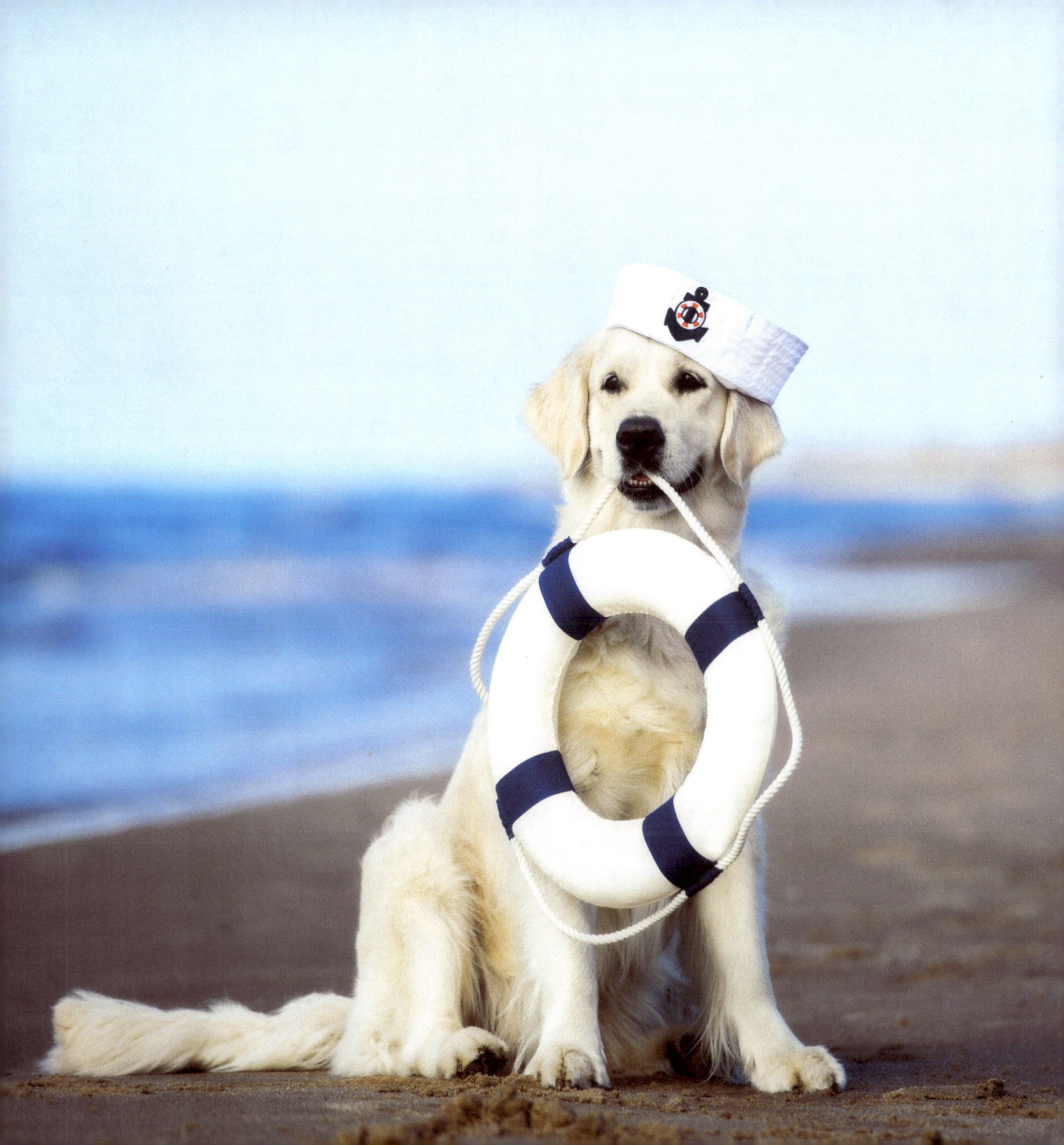

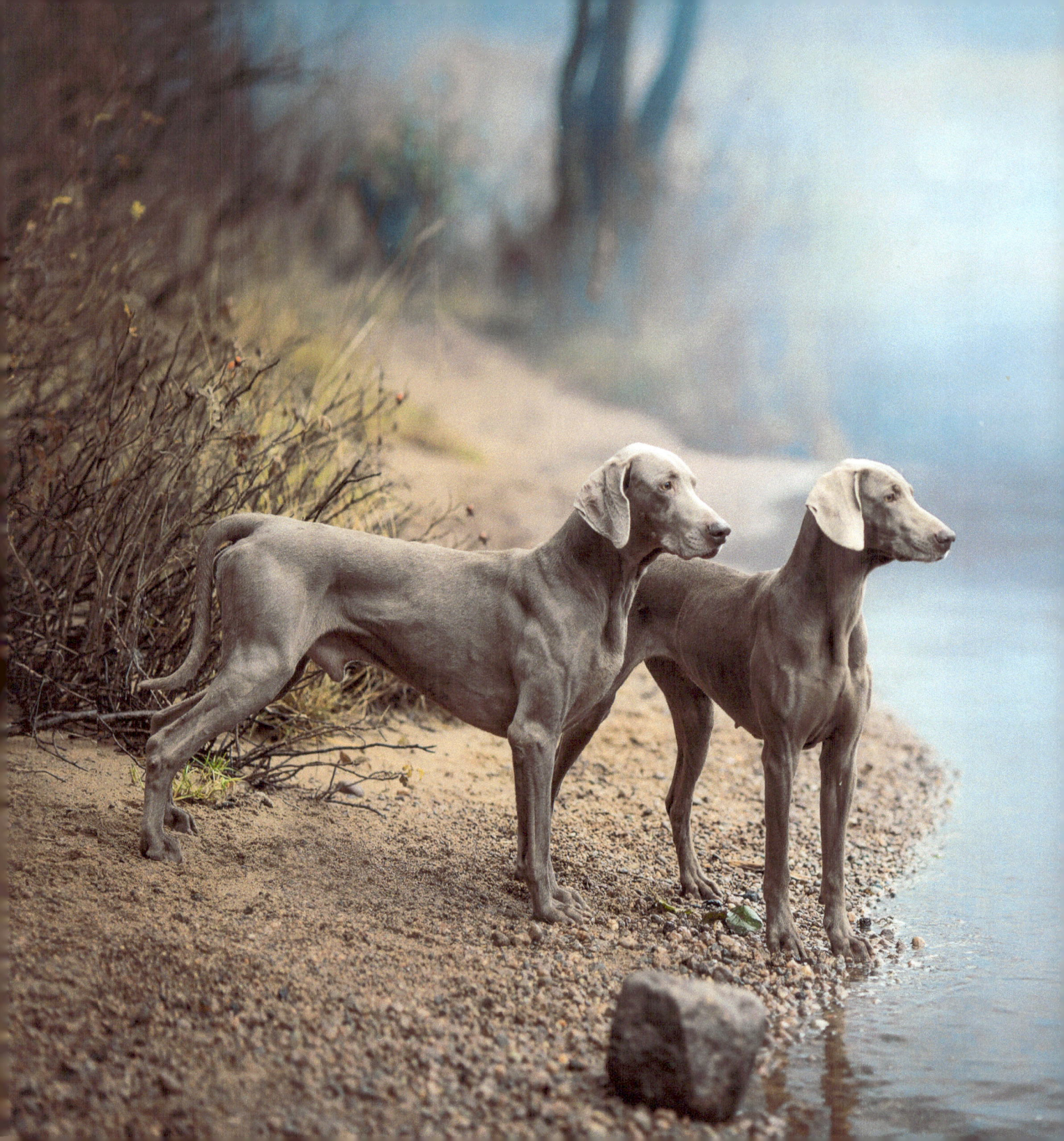

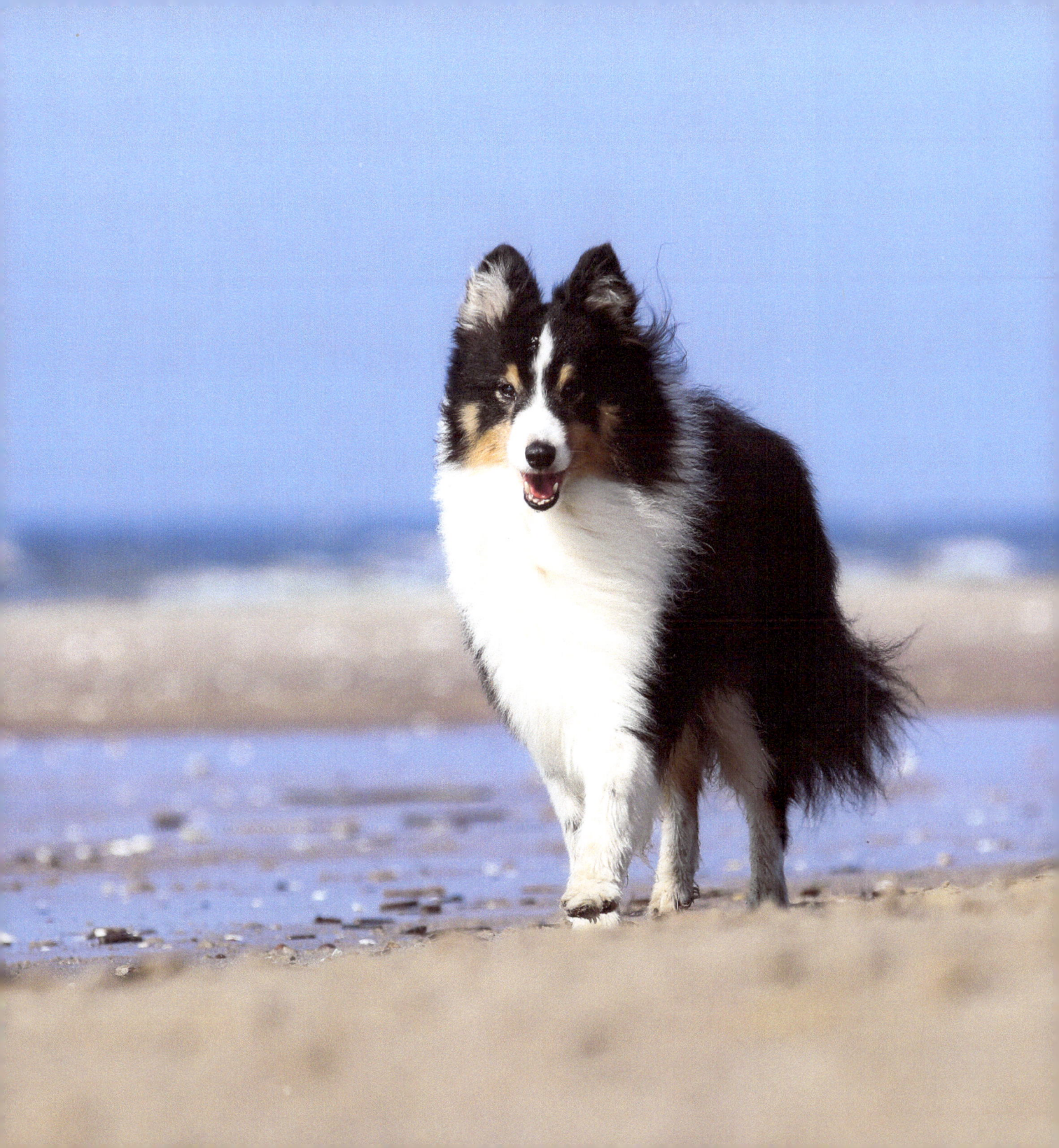

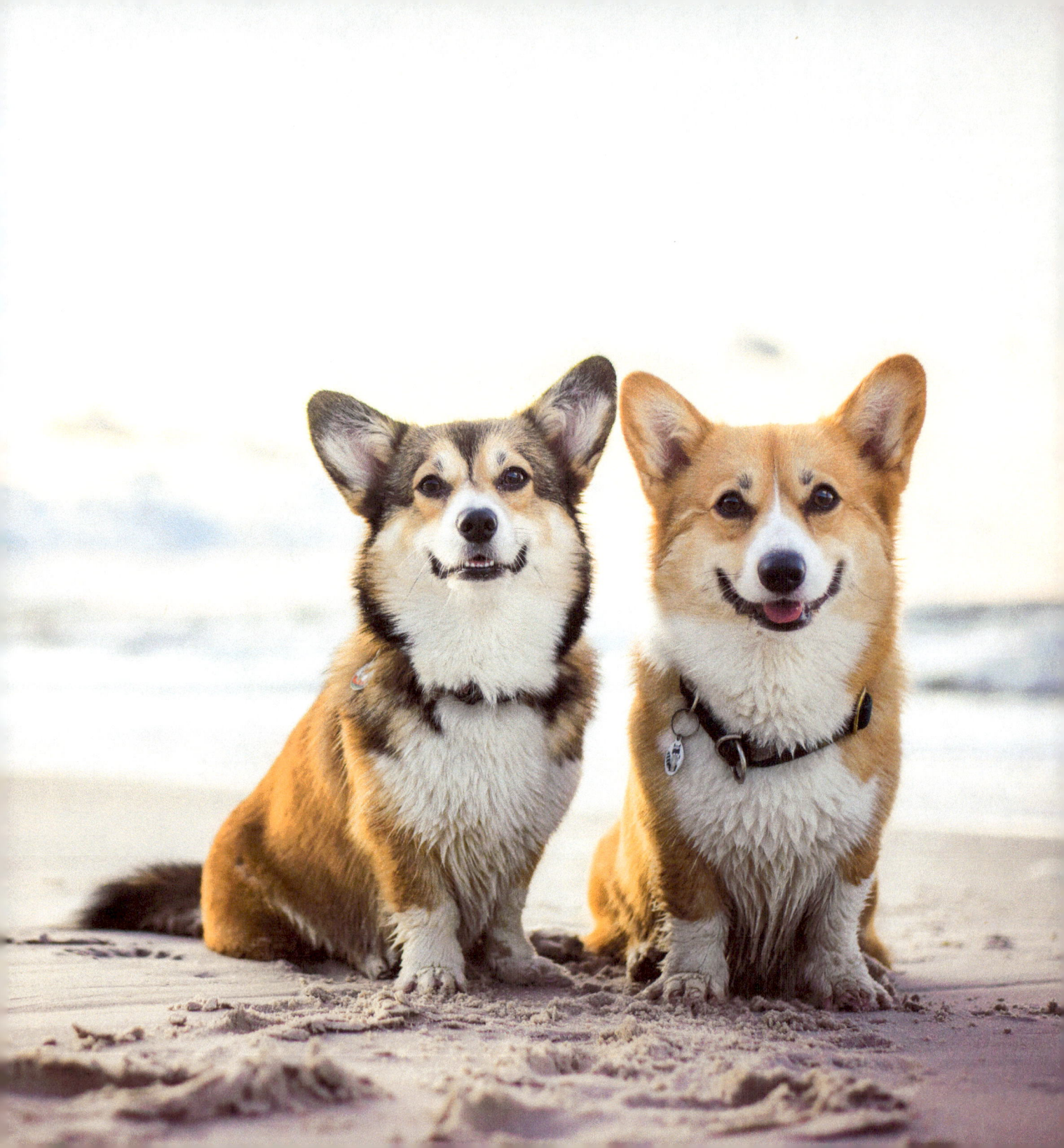

www.ingramcontent.com/pod-product-compliance
Lightning Source LLC
Chambersburg PA
CBHW061142030426

42335CB00002B/75